ADD
10
YEARS
TO YOUR
LIFE

William Campbell Douglass, MD

Rhino Publishing, S.A.

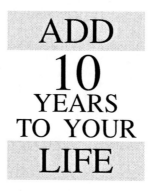

ADD
10
YEARS
TO YOUR
LIFE

Copyright © 1995, 2003
by
William Campbell Douglass, MD

ISBN 9962-636-04-3

Cover illustration by
Alex Manyoma (alex@3dcity.com)

Please, visit Rhino's website for other publications from
Dr. William Campbell Douglass
www.rhinopublish.com

Dr. Douglass' "Real Health" alternative medical
newsletter is available at www.realhealthnews.com

RHINO PUBLISHING, S.A.
World Trade Center
Panama, Republic of Panama
Voicemail/Fax
International: + 416-352-5126
North America: 888-317-6767

Table of Contents

Introduction 1

1   The Resistance Movement 3
2   Racketeering in Medicine 9
3   The Boat That Never Rocks 15

4   Adventures in Iatrogenesis 21
     How Your Doctor Can Kill You 23
     MRI = Mighty Risky Intrusion? 23
     Government, Drug Companies,
          and the Death of Children 24
     Do Tranquilizers Cause Heart Attacks? 25
     Multibillion-Dollar Mistreatment? 26
     Arthritis and the Quack-Busters 28
     Pain — Tell Your Doctor It's Unnecessary 30
     Vasectomy — Safe or Not? 34

5   How to Live a Long Life 39
     Sleeping Without Drugs 41
     Before Cooking Fish, Give It a Hydrogen
     Peroxide Bath 44

6   Is Cancer Preventable? 45
     Risk of Cancer from Pesticides in Food 48
     Prostate Cancer — Leave It Alone 50

7   Estrogen, Fat, and Cancer of the Breast 53

8   **Vitamins in the Cure of**
     Cancer — An Unprecedented Study 59
     Folie Acid — It's About Time 60
9   **Chelation Works!** 63
10 **Salt of the Earth** 73
11 **Hey, Doc! What About...?** 87

Introduction

To add ten years to your life, you need more than just a good doctor. You need to have the right attitude about health and an understanding of the health industry and what it's feeding you. Following the established line on many health issues could make *you* very sick or *worse!*

Take for instance the cardiologist for the Boston Celtics, Dr. W. Thomas Nessa. At 48, he was the picture of health. He followed the line on nutrition, exercise (he ran the Boston Marathon several times), and medical care. That is, until he dropped dead of a heart attack — the very thing he was trained to prevent.

Basically, you've got to take responsibility for your health. In the pages that follow, you'll begin to take the steps necessary to avoid the same fate as Dr. Nessa. And rest assured that, because of the vast amount of misinformation in the health field, we're working hard to provide you with all the "right stuff" to help you live a long, healthy life.

Through the years, my newsletters has helped thousands of people achieve dynamic health and what follows is sort of a "best of" my newsletters. I'm sure you'll find many valuable — and many helpful — items in the pages that follow.

We want you to add *at least* ten years to your life.

William Campbell Douglass, MD
January 1995

Chapter 1

The Resistance Movement

Back in the '60s, and even into the '70s, everyone, including me, thought we had seen the beginning of the end for infectious diseases. The progenitors of penicillin and tetracycline assured us of an unending supply of bug-busters. The war against bacteria was over and done with. But to our great horror the bacteria never surrendered — they went into a resistance movement.

The Resistance Movement began when the staph germ started terrorizing our hospitals with infections that wouldn't respond to antibiotics. We thought Staphylococcus was strictly a skin disease, but in the '50s we started seeing staph pneumonia. One of my intern pals almost died from it. We should have learned a lesson from that, but we knew the pharmaceutical industry with all its chemical miracle-makers wouldn't let us down.

Now hospital staph infections are resistant to all antibiotics but vancomycin. According to Dr. William Pasculle, a microbiologist at the University of Pittsburgh, "The thought of vancomycin resistance getting into something like staph is really frightening."

Most doctors didn't fully realize that the Resistance Movement had become an all-out counterattack until Jim Henson, the creator of the Muppets, died of what would have been considered a simple pneumonia a few years ago. But the situation has become inexorably worse since Henson's tragic death.

The responsibility for this major decline in the effectiveness of antibiotics can largely be placed at the feet of doctors who used antibiotic drugs for 50 years as a shortcut for cures. There is no way of knowing how many hundreds of millions of antibiotic pills and shots were given to patients for the treatment of the common cold, an infection that is self-limiting in over 99 percent of healthy people. Colds and flu do not respond to antibiotics anyway, and may in fact be made worse by their use.

In the past, I have also put some of the blame on the patients for demanding antibiotics from their doctor for every little sniffle, ache, and skin zit that carne along. While this is definitely part of the problem, most of the blame must be placed on a media campaign that has consistently deceived the American people about the true role and ability of antibiotics. But the doctors can't hide behind that excuse, even though they were certainly propagandized more than the patients through such media mouthpieces as the *Journal of the American Medical Association*, and now even the *New England Journal of Medicine*.

Medical students have long been admonished not to use antibiotics for colds and other viral infections. But once set free from the restraints of academia, young doctors rapidly come under the influence of the drug companies, the medical journals beholden to those companies, and the pressure of patients who have been conned into believing that antibiotics are a phylactery of infinite power and goodness.

Let me give you a classic example of what can be done with a little patience and a cooperative patient. I was in Turkey with a friend who developed a terrible case of "the flu" with aching, coughing, and nasal congestion. She got to the point where she was bringing up with her cough and out of her nose a thick, almost dough-like yellow-green discharge. Generally, green means "go" in therapy — go with the antibiotics — because the green color signifies the dreaded Pseudomonas. *Not one doctor in a hundred,* at that point, would resist the urge to prescribe antibiotics for fear of this mighty little creature.

Nine times out of ten that fear is justified, but in this case the temperature was only moderately elevated, the patient was not evidencing any signs of toxicity, and her lungs were perfectly clear. So, although she was coughing up this terrible discharge, it was apparently coming from drainage of the sinuses and not from a bronchial infection or pneumonia. If we could keep the nose draining, and she didn't develop blocked sinuses, I reasoned that we wouldn't have to reach for the antibiotic bottle. I gave her Afrin spray for the sinus discharge and some aspirin (I'm not completely drug-free), and the next day she was 50 percent well. Twenty-four hours later, she had forgotten that she had been sick.

We have seen that common sense is too often neglected and prescriptions are handed out as a first recourse, instead of a last. The result of this gross negligence is a resistance that is quickly spreading from one bacteria to another. Two million people a year now acquire infections, sometimes fatal, after they enter the hospital. Sixty percent of all hospital-acquired infections are resistant to at least one antibiotic and those resistant to *all* drugs are increasing at a frightening rate. Vancomycin, the "drug of last resort," is now in retreat and, according to the Centers for Disease Control, Vancomycin-resistant bacteria in intensive-care wards more than doubled from 1991 to 1992 — and quadrupled the rate of 1990.

Bacteria, even so-called benign ones like the E. coli being used all over the world for genetic engineering, can transfer the genes for antibiotic resistance to other, more aggressive germs. The increasing resistance to Vancomycin is "setting the stage for a more serious health crisis," reports Mike Toner in the *Atlanta Journal.*

As disturbing as this situation is, you will be more disturbed to know that you cannot find out the infection rate of a hospital you are considering using for major surgery. *Hospitals are not required to reveal this information to patients,* and most refuse to do so. A spokeswoman for the University of Pittsburgh Medical Center said: "If we gave people a full list of things they might catch, I don't think anybody would come to a hospital." This generally excellent medical center is a good example of the crisis that is approaching. The university is struggling with a medical nightmare of bacterial infections resistant to all antibiotics.

Hospitals like the University of Pittsburgh have elabórate procedures to avoid bacterial invasions. They have infection-control teams that do nothing but worry about, and take action against, potential areas of breakdown that might lead to infection of patients. But in spite of this complex and very expensive medical bunker, the germs have made a very successful penetration. The university has had 30 cases of infection with an intestinal bacterium resistant to all antibiotics and some of the patients have died. And this is one of the *best* hospitals.

Action to Take

1. Don't be afraid to ask your doctor questions about any drugs or treatment he is prescribing for you. The old saying, "What you don't know won't hurt you," is not always true when it comes to your health.

2. If you are facing surgery, insist that your doctor find out what the infection rate is at that hospital and,

even if it is historically low, if they are currently having any infection problems.

3. If you can afford it, and it is available, ask for a private room in the intensive care unit if you are going to need intensive care.

Ref: *Atlanta Journal and Constitution*, September 19, 1992.

Chapter 2

Racketeering in Medicine

The best definition of medical racketeering I have seen is that of Dr. James P. Carter, author of *Racketeering In Medicine* — *the Suppression of Alternatives:* "The wide-ranging mosaic of special-interest groups who wield undue influence for maximizing profit and perpetuating the status quo in medical fields."

This "mosaic of special-interest groups" includes, of course, the doctors who have allowed themselves to be seduced (or cowed) by the AMA and the PDA. I have called present-day doctors a lot of things, but never "racketeer." But why not? What else would you call someone who uses quack-chemical compounds that don't work and take money for it?

Professor Lowell Levin, Yale University, is even tougher on the medics than Drs. Carter and Douglass: He says that today's licensed physician is more like "some kind of a bug with antennae than a fellow human being." Calling his colleagues cockroaches is *tough*, but, with some notable exceptions, I'm forced to agree with him. Doctors, at least too many of them, have financial reasons for resisting change. If a doctor owns stock in a drug company that produces those deadly "anti-cancer" chemicals, a radiation therapy instrument, or an arthritis drug, is he likely to be enthusiastic about some cheap treatment, such as homeopathy, chelation therapy, or nutritional remedies?

Although we have too many laws on the books, I think it should be illegal for doctors and their families to own stock in the treatments they employ. It's a conflict of interest.

Dr. Carter says: "The financial giants of business ... and their corporate-sponsored philanthropies, such as the American Cancer Society, spend and lobby mightily for laws representing their investments. These forces are intended to maintain the strong financial return on medical investments and to suppress the competition from alternative treatments which might have prevented medicine's financial mess we are faced with today."

Dr. Harris Coulter, medical historian, was the first to point out in his seminal book, *Divided Legacy* (Center for Empirical Medicine, 4221 45th Street, N.W., Washington, D.C. 20016), that the AMA was formed for political reasons, not for the promotion of truth in science and medicine. The homeopathic medical profession was actually beating them out with patient satisfaction — a direct result of non-toxic cures and a personal approach to the patient's problems.

Let's get into the racketeering charge of Dr. Carter so that you can decide if he's (like me) a little obsessed with the rottenness of it all. The NCAHF, the National Council Against Health Fraud, is a front organization for the AMA, the FDA, and the pharmaceutical companies. This group of quacks, a bunch of M.D.s who couldn't cure a carbuncle, are the nexus for the three-headed hydra that will destroy your right to choose the kind of medical care you want. That three-headed snake is the AMA, the government, and the drug industry – the Gang of Three that's determined to crush any opposition to toxic medicine.

David Kessler, FDA commissioner under Bush and one of the few Bush appointees considered extreme left enough to be kept on in the Clinton Administration, is an important enforcer in this vicious troika. He's described by the *Wall Street Journal* as "the archetypical bureaucratic empire builder." That's too kind: He's a slimy and feckless political chameleon out to destroy what's left of freedom of choice in American medicine. The PDA has clearly taken on a KGB complexion since Comrade Kessler took over. Although you are not seeing it in the press, raids by armed PDA goons on health food stores, nutrient manufacturers, and natural healers have become routine. PDA is the attack dog for the drug cartel and the AMA.

The forementioned "private" front for the AMA and the drug industry, the National Council Against Health Fraud (NCAHF), is a strike force which is financed by the AMA, the drug industry, and, covertly, by the federal government. Its purpose is to smash all competition to toxitherapy as practiced by 90 percent of American doctors. Although it is illegal for the federal government to engage in persecuting one group of competitors in order to give advantage to another, Kessler's KGB is involved, full force, and actually runs it. In fact, although it would be denied, there is little doubt that the NCAHF is hooked up to government computers so that the names of counter revolutionaries can be hounded out of practice.

Ironically, this den of jackals is given free rent and the use of the facilities of the Seventh Day Adventist Loma Linda University in California to do its intelligence work and then target these natural medicine practitioners for destruction. The Seventh Day Adventists, who have always championed natural remedies, are now supporting and partially financing its destruction! *[To protest — send letters to Loma Linda University, Loma Linda, CA 92350.]*

The three principle paid stooges of the anti-health conspiracy are Drs. Herbert, Barrett, and Renner. Victor

Herbert is such a fanatic, and makes such a fool of himself in his foaming-at-the-mouth testimony against natural medicine that he is no longer taken seriously. Stephen Barrett is a psychiatrist, so that takes care of his credibility. That leaves John Renner of Kansas City.

Renner is an internist who has set himself up as an expert who passes judgment on what insurance companies should and should not pay. He created the Consumer Health Information Research Institute (CHIRI) and elected himself president. The insurance companies pay Renner to tell them not to pay what they weren't going to pay anyway. In other words, he's a paid mouthpiece of the insurance industry which legitimizes their discrimination against doctors who prefer not to use toxic drugs for treatment of their patients and against those who don't have an AMA ticket. It's known as cartelization and conspiracy — and it stinks.

If Renner and his feeders were to pull this kind of squeeze on any other industry, the airlines for instance, they would be in the Crowbar Hotel in a jiffy. Can you imagine it? "We of the Consumer Flight Information Institute (financed by, let's say, United Airlines) don't like the way you, Delta Airlines, discriminate against minority groups. You hire no Chechens, Azerbaijanis, or Mori Indians, so we have recommended that your liability insurance be cancelled." Would United have the gaul to attempt such a thing? *The insurance industry does it all the time to* defenseless practitioners of biologically-based, non-toxic medicine who don't carry Colt ,45s, stun guns, or dog poison to defend themselves.

Renner admitted under oath that he has a list of 40,000 health providers on his computer that he, Renner, suspects of using "questionable medical practices." Who anointed this gadfly to judge the rest of us? How can you get away with becoming a self-appointed dictator who reports to state medical boards, advising them on whom to sic their regulatory dogs of war, and "advises" insurance companies not to pay for the services of these errant physicians?

Another organization recently brought in to terrorize doctors and insure that they conform is OSHA, the Occupational Safety and Health Administration. Using the excuse that the government needs to protect the patients from blood borne diseases, such as hepatitis and AIDS, OSHA will make unannounced inspections of doctors' offices. They will come without a search warrant and hit the doctor with $1,000 fines like passing out Kleenex. If no effort is made immediately, I mean *immediately*, to correct the violation, the federal sniffer can and will slap the doc with *another* $1,000 hit.

This is clearly unconstitutional, and the courts have so ruled, but these hit teams serve a "higher purpose" — their commissars in Washington. The Association of American Physicians and Surgeons, in a recent issue of their newsletter, *AAPS News*, commented: "This appears to be a methodical takeover of physicians' offices." Henry Thoreau, one of America's greatest freedom fighters put it more quaintly in 1859:

> I went to the store the other day to buy a bolt for our front door, for, as I told the storekeeper, the Governor was coming to the village. "Aye," said he, "and the legislature too."
>
> "Then I will take *two* bolts," said I. He said that there had been a steady demand for bolts and locks of late, for our protectors were coming.

Action to Take

1. Read Dr. Carter's revealing, and disturbing book and, while you are still disturbed about it, ask your con-

gressmen and your senators to hold an investigation into this conspiracy to destroy biologically-based medical practice. Ask him to have his *wife* read the book and report back. Representatives, for the most part, can't read — how else can you account for the way most of them vote?

2. Keep informed of what's going on in the health field by subscribing to the *AAPS News* — $35.00 from the Association of American Physicians and Surgeons, 1601 N.Tucson Blvd., Suite 9, Tucson, AZ 85716.

Chapter 3

The Boat That Never Rocks

Your government operates a department that is vital to your health and well-being that you have probably never heard of. It's called the Division of Biologic Standards (DBS). This agency of approximately 300 people is nestled on the "campus" of the National Institutes of Health in Bethesda, Maryland, and is responsible for assuring the purity and safety of the vaccines doctors jab into you and your little ones.

Has this "watch dog" agency served you well, according to the mandate of your Congress? Or has it, like most government institutions, failed the people and managed to serve only itself? What kind of track record does the division have in fulfilling its regulatory responsibilities? Does its research, financed by you, the taxpayer, have any practical application or is it just another way to milk the taxpayer of his hard-earned dollars?

These questions are not easy to answer because of the secretive, good-old-boy network that controls vaccine quality control in this country. The DBS interlocks with the Centers for Disease Control (Advisory Committee on Immunization Practices) and the Armed Forces Epidemiologic Board. When disaster strikes, such as the typhus vaccine fiasco which was exposed in 1969, the

AFEB can point to the CDC, which can point to the DBS, which can point to the AFEB, and no one ever answers for any wrongdoing.

The boat never rocks at the Division of Biologic Standards because they have built-in safeguards, not against faulty and potentially disastrous vaccines, but against exposure to the public and Congress. The typhus vaccine fiasco mentioned above is a good case in point.

Every army recruit since World War II has been vaccinated against typhus. This was done in spite of the fact that few American soldiers are ever exposed to typhus; the disease is easily controlled in endemic areas by spraying for lice (which transmit the disease) and antibiotics are effective in the treatment of the acute infection.

The mass inoculation of our young men with this foreign animal protein, with unknown long-term effects (more on that later) was a senseless and irresponsible act. But to compound the fiasco, this vaccine, used for twenty-five years, was found in 1969 to be *completely useless* as a protection against typhus. The vaccine had *regularly passed testing by the DBS* and presumably the testing of the Armed Forces Epidemiologic Board and the CDC. Keep in mind that these three boards of medical bureaucrats are responsible for the safety of every shot injected into your children.

A.D. Langmuir, formerly head of the epidemiology branch of the Centers for Disease control, exposed the incompetence and the quackery of the mass annual inoculations against influenza. He said it was a "forcing on the public of a bogus situation.... The vaccine we were promoting was not having any beneficial effects."

The *bad* effects of the vaccine, if any, may not be seen for 30 years and, if they do occur, no one will associate them with the vaccine — or with the DBS, your ever-vigilant watchdog of purity.

The vaccine community is extremely sensitive to the eroding of confidence by the American people in the entire concept of vaccination and the authorities who promote them. So the vaccinators will go to extraordinary lengths to cover up any fiascoes or disasters that may occur, even if their actions are detrimental to the public health. I can assure you they are not as confident in the efficacy and safety of what they do as their often arrogant demeanor would indicate.

This anxiety showed through the bureaucratic mist at one conference on vaccines when the chairman of a National Institutes of Health committee said: "From our debates on what is best or what is wrong, we are conditioning the public to reject measures that sometimes ... are very important." Translation: The public is too stupid, ignorant and skittish to be told the truth about our mistakes and shortcomings. If we rock the boat publically, it might turn over and our whole vaccine package, a hundred years in the making, will go overboard, along with our revered druggist and master promoter, Louie Pasteur.

The most blatant and tragic example of the tendency of these agencies to cover up their mistakes "for the good of the public" was the SV40 scandal of 1961. You may never have heard of this disaster but you or one of your children could die of a brain tumor because of it.

SV40 is the abbreviation of a monkey virus called simian virus 40. Monkey kidney cells were used to make the famous Salk vaccine (that didn't work). The vaccine was contaminated with SV40 and the DBS, the CDC, and the AFEB *all* failed to find it. The vaccine was declared safe and injected into millions of young Americans.

SV40 was found to cause cancer in hamsters, primarily brain tumors, Even though the viral contaminant was found to be cancer-causing, *the DBS and its ex-*

pert advisory committee decided to leave existing stocks of the vaccine on the market rather than risk "eroding public confidence" by a recall.

A recent study in the *American Journal of Medicine* concluded that the number of new cases of brain tumors in Americans under 45 years of age has been mounting at the astounding rate of two percent a year since 1973. If that's compound interest, there are a lot of people walking around with an unwanted lump in their heads directly attributable to bureaucratic incompetence and criminal action.

Some people want to blame electromagnetic radiation from power lines for the skyrocketing incidence of brain tumors, but I have a more 'plausible explanation — and you know what it is.

Ironically, the DBS was established as a result of the original polio disaster in which Salk's improperly tested vaccine, by the Laboratory of Biologic Control (LBC), caused paralytic polio in many of the recipients of the shots.

The transfer of responsibility from the LBC to the DBS is reminiscent of the recent "fall" of the communist states of Eastern Europe. The communist bosses of many of these countries merely changed their label from communist to capitalist and still run their fiefdoms as before. The director and the laboratory chief of LBC stayed on at DBS and so the only change was the name. More and bigger disasters were inevitable.

The DBS is supposed to be a research organization as well as a regulatory body. But, because of the anti-boat-rocking mentality of the bureaucratic scientists in charge, nothing much happens and scientific initiative is quickly punished and suppressed. J. Anthony Morris, a research scientist at DBS, raised questions about the efficacy of the influenza vaccine. He was promptly transferred.

An even more shocking case of disregard for the public welfare, and suppression of scientific findings that affected millions of Americans, was the report by a DBS scientist that the SV40 viral contaminant in the polio vaccine caused cancer in hamsters. He was *demoted!*

A DBS research contractor discovered that the dog kidney cells to be used for the manufacture of rubella vaccine were contaminated with a herpes virus. When this was brought to the attention of the DBS authorities, they chose not to investigate the matter further. Does the rubella vaccine used today contain a herpes contaminant? I don't know and I doubt that DBS knows, or cares — as long as no one rocks the DBS boat.

In light of the AIDS epidemic and the fact that the virus was most likely of laboratory origin, the lead paragraph in an article from *Science* magazine was more prophetic than the author could have ever imagined. Editor Wade Nichols said 20 years ago:

"There can be few graver opportunities for manmade disaster than the mass immunization campaigns that are now routine in many countries. Should the vaccine preparations become contaminated with an undetected agent ... such as a cancer-causing virus, *a whole generation of [vaccinated people] could be put in jeopardy.*

"This, of course, is no science fiction writer's horror story — *it has already happened once* millions of people have been injected with a monkey virus ... which was found to be contaminating polio vaccines. The virus causes cancer in hamsters; no one yet knows what it may do in man." (Emphasis added.)

Action to take:

Show this chapter to your congressman and ask him if anybody in Congress is checking on these scientists who are responsible for the purity of these vaccines. They insist that you must submit your children to their sacred rites of exorcism of certain evil germs but their record of control of contaminants is not as good as their record of control of the American people.

Ref: *Science*, March 17, 1972, pp. 1225-1230.

Chapter 4

Adventures in Iatrogenesis

Iatrogenesis means injury to the patient caused by the doctor. This problem is immense and you need to be aware of it. Iatrogenic events are an inevitable concomitant of technological progress. As medicine becomes more complicated, more mistakes are being made. There are just more variables than a human can handle. There have been, for instance, about 5,000 new pharmaceutical preparations marketed in the past decade. Many of these are merely variations of other drugs, which adds to the confusion. One study revealed that iatrogenic events occur in 19.2 percent of hospitalized patients, half of those due to therapeutic drugs. *(Hospital Practice*, January 30, 1989).

The iatrogenic injury I am going to describe to you is far more common than realized and is absolutely inexcusable. During this flu season, you could become a victim of the same type of illogical and irresponsible medicine.

Pat, a 50-year-old female, came down with the flu. She went to her "highly respected and well-trained" internist for treatment. He did what many doctors do, in spite of the fact that scores of scientific studies have shown that it doesn't work. He gave her antibiotics for her viral infection.

She recovered in about ten days which is about the time you would expect to be sick without any treatment at all. A few weeks later, she developed a high fever, back pain, and pain on urination. Tests revealed a kidney infection called pyelonephritis. This is no longer a common infection and, in her case, was probably caused by a depression of her immune system due to the antibiotics.

Pat was admitted to the hospital where she received even more powerful antibiotics intravenously which were necessary due to the seriousness of the kidney infection. So a case of the flu, for which there is no known conventional therapy, was turned into a kidney infection and a $2,000 hospital stay.

As doctors, we should try to do the best we can for our patients and not give them prescriptions simply because the patient expects them. A basic principle taught in medical school is "beneficence": One must work to contribute to the well-being of the patient. If circumstances make this impossible, beneficence dictates that we be honest with the patient and tell them that Father Time and Mother Nature, beings which only God controls, must be relied upon for a cure. Tell the patient that the medication, if any, that you are prescribing is for comfort and not for cure. Many doctors don't do this and thus steal the credit from God. Remember that old saying: "God heals; the doctor collects the fee." Sometimes, God heals in spite of the doctor, such as in the case above.

The other principle guiding physicians is that of "nonmaleficence": Avoid doing harm to the patient. This principle goes back at least to Hippocrates who said in his oath for physicians: "First, do no harm."

Action to take:

If you ever contract the flu, and there is a strong possibility that you will, refuse antibiotics unless the doctor can give you a clear reason for taking them. Having a viral infection, the flu, is not an indication for antibiotics.

How Your Doctor Can Kill You

If you have a heart attack, this information could save your life — *if your* doctor acts on it. The problem is that he probably will not, as most doctors refuse to accept the mountain of evidence that has proven magnesium can save your life if given promptly following a heart attack. Magnesium reduces the death rate from myocardial infarction by as much as 90 percent.

This means if you don't get magnesium following a heart attack, and you are tissue-deficient in magnesium, *you are nine times more likely to die if you have the wrong doctor.* Ask your doctor if he understands the role of magnesium in heart attacks and if he would administer it to you if you had one. If he says no, and you are over 60, I would consider finding a doctor who understands this important therapy.

Your doctor may try, in fact almost certainly will try, to "snow" you with glowing reports on the clot-busters now being employed for acute heart attacks. You can startle him by replying: "I understand streptokinase and TPA can induce a stroke from bleeding in the brain and is quite expensive, whereas magnesium is quite safe and very cheap. Would you read these articles about magnesium and then discuss this with me again?"

Give him the following references:

South African Medical Journal, 1958;32:1211
Medical Proc, 1959;5:487
Lancet, 1986:1:234
American Journal of Cardiology, 1990:66:271-274

MRI = Mighty Risky Intrusion?

The MRI, magnetic resonance imaging, has been a great advance in diagnosis as it gives incredibly sharp pictures of the internal organs. But like all high-energy technology, there are dangers. Thermal injuries from the procedure, ranging from minor burns to extensive third-degree burns requiring skin grafts have occurred and even fires in the magnetic bore have been reported. There have been two deaths reported in patients with pacemakers.

The problem, one investigator said, is probably much worse than it appears as only the most severe injuries are being reported. The number of these scans is increasing by tens of thousands each year and so it is likely that this new iatrogenic injury will soon make the front pages of America's newspapers.

Ref: *Internal Medicine News*, October 15-31, 1990

Government, Drug Companies, and the Death of Children

At least 1,470 children have died from Reye's syndrome because of government incompetence and pharmaceutical company callousness. After it was proven that aspirin caused the disease, it took bureaucrats *five years* to get around to requiring aspirin manufacturers to put warning labels on the product. Of course, aspirin manufacturers could have put the labels on without being required to do so, but *that* would have cost money.

Both organizations knew that the use of aspirin to treat the flu and chicken pox causes Reye's syndrome, which induces lethargy, coma, and death in children. Isn't there any way we can punish the government and drug companies? They certainly punish us a lot.

Ref: *International Herald Tribune*, October 24-25, 1992.

Do Tranquilizers Cause Heart Attacks?

From the University of Oxford comes a report that will give the psychiatrists something else to be depressed about. All of the mood-altering drugs - anti-depressants, tranquilizers, mood-elevators, whatever you want to call them - have been found to be related to a higher incidence of fatal heart attacks in women. This finding is independent of other risk factors, such as smoking or previous heart disease. Of great significance is that this association with cardiac death is stronger with *current use* of the drugs, although there is also correlation, although weaker, with previous use of these mind-benders.

Even more startling is that the subjects were all *young women*, between the ages of 16 and 39. The relationship of tranquilizers to fatal heart attacks in older women, or men of any age, has not been investigated and, because of these alarming findings, there is an urgent need for such an investigation.

The study also revealed *a threefold increase in subarachnoid hemorrhage* with the use of psychotropic drugs. This was not as strong a correlation as that of a fatal heart attack but is still impressive. The rate of increased cardiac death in patients taking the drugs was *seventeenfold!*

Militating against the relationship of cardiac death and tranquilizers is the observation that the correlation is present no matter which class of drug is prescribed. How can drugs with different mechanisms of action cause the same pathology, i.e., fatal heart attacks? This, of course, is not impossible and may be more a measure of our ignorance of the mechanism used by these drugs.

Action to take: Psychiatric problems seem to have become more prevalent with the advent of these drugs, starting with Thorazine in the 1950s. The action to take would seem obvious - *don't take these dangerous drugs.* Take a walk, talk to a friend, have a cup of tea, go to church. My friend, Major Ramsey Tainsh, Indian Army, Retired, disarmed entire native armies in Burma with nothing but warm tea (with sugar) and a little cajoling.

Multibillion-Dollar Mistreatment?

Are the wonder drugs for the treatment of peptic ulcer really that wonderful? According to a British doctor, not only are they *not* wonderful, they are the *wrong treatment.*

We have had many letters asking about the safety and effectiveness of the anti-ulcer drugs Tagamet and Zantac. "My long-suffering husband," one subscriber writes, "has been taking Zantac for a year and a half. He ran out of pills, but is thinking of ordering more. He has no ulcer now, as far as we know, but he is still unable to eat certain foods, such as tomatoes, yet he can take beer and soda pop. Will the Zantac prevent the recurrence of the ulcer?" (L.F., Oklahoma)

The Glaxo Corporation was called on the carpet recently in England for exaggerating the effectiveness of Zantac to doctors. If you have read my monograph, *Dangerous (Legal) Drugs,* you know that Tagamet, the other superstar in the ulcer field, can kill you if you become exposed to certain pesticides while taking the drug.

The amount of money — and waste of precious funds — involved here is colossal. Zantac is the best-selling drug in the world and people spend, world-wide, *five billion dollars* yearly on ulcer drugs. Many people have to take these expensive pharmaceuticals for life, but they get recurrences of the ulcer anyway. It's hard to imagine that people can be so taken in these days by such an international phoney medicine-man show — really little different from the snake-oil hucksters of the nineteenth Century, only electronic and telephonic.

When you add to this chicanery the toxicity of the drugs and the simple fact that these drugs give only *temporary relief* and *do not prevent recurrence*, as the companies have implied (there is a 90 percent recurrence rate), then it's time to look for more effective means of therapy.

We've mentioned Duopept, the remarkable, nontoxic treatment from South Africa, but it's not available in the U.S. anymore; the drug companies had their puppets in the PDA outlaw it. However, there is a treatment that goes directly to the problem and it will no doubt surprise you: antibiotic therapy. We reported years ago on the finding that peptic ulcer had been found to be a bacterial infection of the lining of the stomach or duodenal wall caused by Helicobacter pylori.

A treatment of a broad-spectrum antibiotic for three weeks will cure 95 percent of ulcers *without recurrence.* Doctors have ignored this treatment because of the incessant propaganda by the drug companies for the ulcer drugs, ignorance of the scientific literature, timidity about trying something new (the discovery of H. pylori was over ten years ago), and, as British gastroenterologist Kenneth McColl says, "prescribing inertia."

Antibiotics are overused and misused, yes, but here is a clear indication for them that can save billions of dollars worldwide. An even better solution, however, would probably be the use of photoluminescence therapy. As you know, antibiotics can lead to serious complications; phototherapy does not. I don't know of any case studies using photoluminescence for peptic ulcer, but infection is infection and it should work effectively. But if doctors won't use a simple antibiotic therapy, how long will it be before they use photoluminescence?

Arthritis and the Quack-Busters

Let me say right up front, as I have many times in the past, that there is no known cure for rheumatoid arthritis - and that includes any drug your rheumatologist may prescribe for you. In fact, the very hypocrisy of the medical establishment I've tried to warn you about in these pages is running rampant in the field of rheumatology. As with psychiatry and psychology, rheumatology, the treatment of rheumatoid arthritis, is a field where the practitioners *know* their treatment doesn't work, but still take their patients' hard-earned money for their "therapy."

Even though these "conventional" treatments don't work at all, there are many unconventional treatments, some "natural" and some not, that have been found to give dramatic relief from arthritis. Some of these are: EDTA chelation therapy (see Chelation Works! chapter), photo-oxidation (see my book *Into the Light,* available from Rhino Publishing, www.rhinopublish.com), the drug metronidazole (which is effective on those cases caused by an amoebic infestation of the joint), fasting and/or the elimination of foods to which the patient is allergic. There are no doubt others that I don't know about (and I'm sure I'll get a flood of letters on it from which I will probably learn a lot).

An interesting statistic that the Arthritis Foundation would prefer that you didn't know is that ten years after beginning treatment with cortisone, gold injections, and other costly and toxic pharmaceuticals, almost *none* of the patients are still taking the drugs. Wallace V. Epstein, professor of medicine at the University of California, San Francisco (UCSF), has gone so far as to say that *none* of these drugs have been proven to do more good than harm. Moreover, a recent international medical congress in Europe proposed that none of the so-called arthritis drugs should be classified as effective!

Kenneth E. Sack, also from UCSF medical school, took umbrage with Dr. Epstein, but his umbrage ended as a whimper. He made some astonishing revelations and admitted that:

1. none of the anti-arthritis drugs had been proven to alter the course of the disease,

2. the natural history of the disease, i.e., what happens if the disease is left untreated, is still unknown,

3. some patients get better without treatment (or from self-treatment?), and

4. *he has never seen a complete remission of the disease from his therapy.*

Which would you prefer, a "quack remedy" that often works without side effects or an PDA-approved drug that has been proven *not* to work, *by the rheumatologists' own admission,* and may have lethal side effects?

I'll let you decide who the real quacks are.

Action to Take

1. Avoid rheumatologists. They, like the psychiatrists and the cancer chemotherapists, are a danger to your health and well-being. Their results put them well out of the credibility range.

2. Find a practitioner who deals in holistic medicine. The American College of Advancement in Medicine (ACAM) is your best bet. I feel that with arthritis, you have to match the cure to the patient and the answer is rarely drugs, which is all the arthritis specialist knows. To request a free list of doctors, send a SASE with $.55 postage to ACAM, Box 3427, Laguna Hills, CA 92654.

Ref: Gaby, *Townsend Letter for Doctors,* March 1993.

Pain — Tell Your Doctor It's Unnecessary

If you've had surgery, you know all about pain. But did you know that most of the pain suffered by patients is entirely unnecessary, and is due to the ignorance of doctors concerning the proper use of narcotics?

The war on drugs has engendered a neglect of patients in chronic pain. The doctors, fearing that they will be labeled drug-pushers, and suspecting every patient asking for pain relief to be an addict, have abandoned many patients to a life of unremitting pain. This is a great tragedy and is not consistent with the doctor's Hippocratic oath to relieve suffering.

Dr. David Friedman of the National Institute of Drug Abuse, addressing the morality and the ethicality of treating patients in pain, said: "You need not fear that they will become addicted because, almost inevitably, they will not. You must keep compassion foremost in your mind." Many studies have shown that nonaddictive patients — most of us — will not suffer from addiction no matter how much narcotic is given after a painful operation.

At a meeting of the American Pain Society, pain expert Russell Portenoy of the Sloan-Kettering Cancer Center, remarked: "There has been an increasing hysteria about substance abuse in this country.... This tends to have an adverse effect on the appropriate subscribing of narcotic drugs for painful medical conditions."

I had an iatrogenic (doctor-induced) injury to my right wrist that caused a neurological condition called reflex sympathetic dystrophy. An orthopedist did an exploratory operation to the palm of my hand and promised me — absolutely, positively — that he would leave an order for intravenous narcotic to prevent postoperative pain. He forgot to order it and I suffered terribly for the first 12 hours following the surgery. My orthopedist was a nice, gentle, and caring person, but doctors just don't take pain seriously — unless it's their own.

Doctors also have a built-in resistance to giving adequate narcotic therapy for pain: We are taught in medical school that the patient may die of respiratory depression if we don't keep the dose below what he actually needs for relief of his pain. This has been proved *not* to be the case, and patients in severe pain can tolerate large doses of narcotics without compromising their respiration. The body, by mechanisms unknown, can accept larger doses of narcotics when they are needed without danger. Certainly when patients are on intensive care and being observed constantly, there is no excuse for not giving adequate narcotic medication for pain rather than the minimal dose that will keep the patient from screaming or moaning too loudly.

With modern narcotic management, there is absolutely no reason for a patient to experience excruciating pain. Pain expert, Stratton Hill, M.D., said: "As long as the patient is in pain, you really don't have to worry about respiratory depression."

The situation had become so intolerable in Texas that Dr. Hill got a bill passed to protect doctors from the zeal of the state medical board. The board can no longer tell the doctor how much narcotic he can administer to a patient in intractable pain, and he can't be censored for giving these desperate patients all the narcotic they need to avoid suffering.

Seems odd that such a bill should have to be passed, but such is the present atmosphere about drug abuse — the issue is being used to restrict everyone's freedom. So much so that the "war on drugs" is bleeding over into the practice of medicine, making life for many patients absolutely miserable. I'm not sure a war that hurts the good guys so badly is a wise use of money. What do you think?

This underuse of narcotics almost approaches the level of criminal neglect in the case of terminally ill patients. Why in the world should a patient dying of AIDS or cancer be denied all the narcotic he wants and needs to keep him comfortable? The answer often given is that a tolerance will be built up, and then, no matter how much narcotic is given, the patient will not get relief. In other words, the patient needs to suffer now, so that in the long run, he will not have to suffer more as the disease progresses.

But it has been proven that this argument is simply not valid. Studies have shown that maintaining dope addicts on a progressively higher "maintenance dose" of narcotic does not produce a consequent lack of effect from the drug. Many people suffer unnecessary pain because of doctors' lack of understanding of these principles of narcotic therapy.

In regulation-plagued Germany, the government has just about put doctors out of the pain-relieving business. For narcotics, the doctors have to use a triplicate form and fill it out in an exact manner — or else. Exceeding the maximum dose allowed by the bureaucracy is a *criminal act that will land you in jail.* No wonder half of Germany's physicians don't even request the forms — it isn't worth the risk — leaving the patients to suffer. As Ronald Reagan used to say: "Government isn't the solution; government is the problem."

A time-honored method for relieving chronic pain is the use of an anesthetic, such as procaine, as a nerve block. This method may give temporary relief but is seldom curative and, in time, loses its effectiveness. The only type of nerve block that can give permanent relief is the sphenopalatine ganglion block. This treatment has an interesting history and illustrates the hysteria relating to narcotics today that is causing millions of patients to suffer unnecessarily.

The treatment consists of putting Q-tips soaked in cocaine up the nose to rest against the back wall of the throat. Behind that area is the sphenopalatine ganglion, the "switching station" or terminus where *all pain fibers* pass to the brain. When you have surgery, the pain message from the incision must go through this neural highway to get to the pain center of the brain. If this message is blocked, *pain anywhere in the body,* from the big toe to the top of the head, can be relieved. The sphenopalatine ganglion block is very effective at blocking this message.

Strangely, blocking the sphenopalatine ganglion is often curative. In other words, the blockage of the pain is permanent. As an example, back pain is often relieved with this method and it is the treatment of choice for headaches and relieving the pain of severe burns. And, as mentioned earlier in this monograph, addiction is a *non-problem* with these suffering people. I know of no reasonable scientific explanation for such a remarkable phenomenon, but it's true. I used this form of pain treatment on my patients for ten years with great success.

For reasons not understood, increased oxygenation increases the effectiveness of the block. So the therapy should be even more effective if combined with intravenous hydrogen peroxide and photoluminescence, both of which increase the oxygenation of tissues. But you will not find this combination of therapies anywhere in the U.S.

One of my most impressive cases was that of a banker's wife who had suffered from migraine headaches for most of her life. After six treatments, each one painless and taking about 30 minutes, she was completely free of her headaches for the first time in 20 years.

But overregulation, drug paranoia, and bureaucratic zealotry have taken this therapy away from us. If a doctor orders medicinal cocaine for his office today, he will have federal and state narcs at his office the following morning. And because of the "war on drugs," the price of medicinal cocaine has soared to over $1,000 an ounce!

Can you imagine doctors being in a position where government bureaucrats dictate how much human suffering the doctors are allowed to relieve — which is their primary mission as physicians? If Congress ever passes anything like the Clinton health plan, this deplorable and frightening situation will get even worse. Your new medical managers in Washington will not only have the over-zealous "war on drugs" as an excuse to limit human suffering through the restriction of narcotics, but will have the added weapon of "cost containment," which is far more important to them than the fact that you are dying an agonizing death.

Action to Take

1. Prior to surgery, have a friendly discussion with the doctor about pain control and give him a copy of this article. Be sure to underline the quotes from the pain experts.

2. While in the hospital, don't be shy about asking for pain relief.

Vasectomy — Safe or Not?

As the anti-people movement prods us towards birth control, one of the most popular medical subjects has become vasectomy. The following letter is somewhat of a composite of many letters that I have received from my subscribers. These are important questions which many subscribers are wondering about. And these questions need important answers.

Dear Dr. Douglass,

We have three children and want no more. My husband is considering a vasectomy as a permanent solution to the problem. We want to know if it's safe. We have heard that there are risks of heart disease, cancer of the prostate, and of my husband's libido decreasing as well as a decrease in the amount of his ejaculate. I even heard that the operation might cause an enlargement of the prostate which would bring difficulty with urination.

All of this sounds pretty grim and so I am considering a hysterectomy. What do you suggest?

The first thing I would advise is don't have a hysterectomy just as a method of birth control. Although it wouldn't be as foolish as your husband having an "amputation" as a birth-control measure, it is in the same category of unacceptable alternatives.

Many studies on the effects of vasectomy were done through telephone interviews of patients who supposedly had endured one. I say "supposedly" because you would be amazed to know how little people know about their bodies *or what has been done to it* \ For example, a study was done to determine if men knew whether or not they had been circumcised. That may sound like a ridiculous research project for something so obvious and personal, but the results were amazing. About 35 percent of the men turned out to be wrong in their answers. This indicates that reports by patients as to whether or not they have had a vasectomy would be worthless, and so the studies would be equally worthless.

Liver tumors in rats have been clearly demonstrated following vasectomy, but it is impossible to extrapolate this finding to humans. Cardiovascular disease has been reported to be higher in men who have had a vasectomy, but other studies indicate the opposite. So, the jury is still out.

In humans, various types of anti-sperm antibodies have been demonstrated in the blood following vasectomy. Although not a factor in females, some scientists theorize that these anti-sperm antibodies may play an important role in the pathology of AIDS in males. This is not to imply that a man will contract AIDS from his own anti-sperm antibodies following vasectomy, but these foreign antibodies may be a very important factor in AIDS among sodomites. It is also possible that these antibodies, produced following vasectomy, could lead to some type of autoimmune disease later in life, such as arthritis or MS. That is pure speculation on my part and the wielders of the knife and knot will be quick to point out there are no studies demonstrating that undesirable outcome. Their point is correct, but there have been *no* studies to investigate this possibility!

Morphologic changes, i.e., fibrosis, have been well documented following vasectomy. The authors of these reports, according to one leading expert in this field, "argue convincingly" that the visible fibrotic changes result from "mechanical obstruction" and not from any autoimmune effects.

There is often a decrease in the volume of the ejaculate following the surgery, but the size of the gland does not appear to be affected, i.e., there is no enlargement of the prostate as a result of the operation. There is conflicting evidence as to the effect of the procedure on the levels of the male hormone, testosterone.

Back to vasectomy and its relation to prostate cancer: All of the six published studies which addressed the issue of vasectomy and prostate cancer relied upon evidence from self-reports, usually gathered over the phone. So, taking into consideration what we will call the "circumcision phenomenon," misrepresentation is quite plausible and the results of the study could be greatly skewed — in either direction, meaning there is a clear relation between vasectomy and cancer or there clearly is not. Since the vasectomy/cancer relationship is still unknown, I would have to advise against having one until some reliable studies are performed.

If there is an association between prostatectomy and cancer, it is extremely weak. There are other variables associated with prostatic cancer that are far more significant: a father or brother with prostate cancer, cigarette smoking, a history of prostatitis, and a history of an enlarged prostate.

Men who have had a prostatectomy are more prone to inflammation and infection of the epididymis (the gland around the prostate) and inflammation of the testicles than men whose prostates are intact.

When I first began my response to these letters on vasectomy, and before I had completed my review of the literature, I was pretty sure I would end up recommending vasectomy as a safe method of birth control. But after reading the latest articles on the subject, and reading between the lines of those articles, I have reversed myself — and another set of letters has metamorphosed into a polemic, this time against a sacred cow of surgery — the "harmless" vasectomy.

Action to Take

1. Avoid all of the surgical permanent solutions —
vasectomy, tubal ligation, hysterectomy, and mutilation. They are all unacceptable, in my opinion.

2. The healthiest contraception is probably, and pardon me if this sounds a little Ann Landersish, to watch your calendar for your "fun days." If you don't understand what I am saying, then you'd best not try it.

3. The next best method from the standpoint of health would be the diaphragm or cervical cap. There is, though, a risk of infection from both of these methods.

4. I am opposed to the Pill in any variety, including the new one that does your abortion for you (RU486). This new European wonder Pill will revolutionize the birth control industry. It may be safe, but don't bet on it.

Ref: *Contraception*, 1972;5:269-78.
   Immunology of the Male Reproductive System,
      (New York: Marcel Dekker, 1987:171-201).
   New England Journal of Medicine, 1985; 313:1252-1256.
   The Prostate, 1988; 13:57-67.
   Fertility and Sterility, 1988; 49:309-315.
   American Journal of Epidemiology, 1990; 132:1051-1055.
   American Journal of Epidemiology, 1990; 132:1056-1061.
   British Journal of Cancer, 1988; 57:326-331.
   Journal of the American Medical Association, 1984; 252:1023-
      1029.

Chapter 5

How to Live a Long Life

The University of Georgia did a study of centenarians to determine their secrets of a long life. This was one of the best studies of this age group to date, as it didn't take the elderly in their entirety, but concentrated on those who had reached an advanced age and were still mentally alert and active in their community. You will be surprised at what they found and what they did *not* find in this group of 37,000 Americans (that number itself came as a surprise to me).

Every species has a limit to its life span that doesn't vary much, barring war and pestilence. Most birds don't live long, yet parrots can live to the age of 20 or more. Horses have a moderate life span, yet donkeys seem to live forever. People usually don't make it beyond 70 or 80, but more of them are living up to a hundred — though that group is still a distinct minority. In spite of all the medical advances, we seem to reach a cliff at about a hundred years of age where the stubborn remnant of oldsters, after having outlived their children, fall off. So the mortality curve has been pushed to the right, bunching a lot of people up at 80 to 100 but there aren't many folks beyond that point.

I have an ex-relative who does everything wrong. She smokes two packs of cigarettes a day and is drunk every night. She is in her mid-seventies and still functions during the day. Others I have known did everything they were supposed to do in order to stay healthy but died in their prime. I have had friends in their thirties and forties die of asthma, brain tumor, heart attacks, and stroke. They all led relatively healthy lives, as far as I could tell.

Back in 1981, when these senior citizens were youngsters of only 87 or so, a black woman from south Georgia was interviewed for TV on her 105th birthday. When asked the inevitable question, "To what do you owe your long life?", she replied: "I drinks 12 cups of black coffee a day."

One of our subscribers, K.B., another black woman from Georgia wrote in: "I am never sick with no aches or pains." She then described a fainting spell (called syncope, in medical terminology) she had experienced that landed her in the hospital for three days. "They called it syncope. I don't know nothing about syncope. Please tell me about syncope and how to avoid it." She then mentioned, offhandedly, that she was 97 years old! Maybe the answer to longevity is to be black, female and from Georgia — it's a pretty nice place.

In answer to K.B.'s question, we doctors have absolutely nothing to offer for syncope of the elderly (a common complaint). You have probably learned the hard way not to squat (it causes a poorly-understood circulatory reaction and dizziness that can lead to syncope), not to stand up too abruptly, and not to run up the stairs — you weren't born yesterday. Don't let them sell you on surgery to your neck arteries and don't take Antivert, Cyclospasmol, or any other of their toxic placebos. Let *your doctor* take these nostrums — and you'll outlive him.

Although the Georgia researchers worked hard at their study, spending as many as 26 hours talking with an oldster, they didn't come to any hard conclusions. One surprising non-finding was that genetics could not be proven to be an overwhelming factor in longevity. The

Wall Street Journal reported: "Most aging experts (sic — I think they mean experts on aging, but then the experts probably *are* aging) say genetics has a, great deal to do with how long you live." But, the aging experts found, the elderly didn't necessarily have parents or grandparents who had lived long lives. Many of them had also outlived their children, which doesn't say much for the genetics theory.

This demoting of genetics as a major factor in longevity would appear to be good news as it implies there are things we can do to promote a long, healthy life. (I was beginning to wonder.)

One finding of special interest to us flaming carnivores is that a low-animal-fat diet will not cause you to live longer. Most of the oldsters ate bacon, sausage, eggs, and all those other animal foods your doctor says are going to kill you. A "nutrition researcher," commenting on this finding, said that she *still* would recommend low-fat diets, because the fact that these folks had eaten their way to a long healthy life was "probably just a reflection of their cultural upbringing."

Now how is *that* for a non sequitur?

Ref: *Wall Street Journal*, November 12, 1992.

Sleeping Without Drugs

How can being unconscious be so enjoyable? "I slept like a stone — didn't even dream — it was great." There aren't many things as satisfying as a good night's unconsciousness. Why is that? Is life just a fantasy? Is the unconscious state the *real* thing? I suppose not, as consciousness isn't all that bad either — at least for some people. But some of us, at least part of the time, (I'm writing this at three o'clock in the morning) have difficulty achieving that delicious state of morpheus known as sleep.

Are drugs the answer for better sleep? You know how I feel about *that* and now there is good news for us insomniacs, or so the sleep experts claim.

I read an article in the *International Herald Tribune* recently that was headlined: "How to Sleep Without Pills." I thought, "Oh boy, are my readers going to like this." The article was so trite it almost put me to sleep: Worry can keep you awake; relaxation training will help; stress can cause sleeplessness, etc. All of this psychological stuff may be true but is a psychological tune-up the answer to insomnia? I don't think so.

I suspect the answer lies somewhere in the field of electro-medicine, photobiology, magnetic fields or some combination of these forces.

There is now even a journal on sleep, and the lack thereof, called *SLEEP* (it's also a good soporific). The experts on sleep are on to the futility (and danger) of sleeping pills. Dr. Charles Morin of the Sleep Disorders Center, Medical College of Virginia, said: "Sleeping pills are self-limiting in their long-term effectiveness." And, if you have read my monograph on *Dangerous Drugs*, you know that efficacy isn't the only problem with "sleepers" — they can put you to sleep for good.

Dr. Morin has done a study comparing non-drug techniques of sleep induction with sleeping pills. He claims those using his "behavioral methods" reduced their time before falling asleep to 50 minutes as compared to 75 minutes for those who took a sleeper. I am not very impressed with those statistics. There is probably a strong placebo effect, which won't last, and also the please-the-doctor-with-a-favorable-report syndrome (we should have a name for that.)

Most doctors are sticking to the old prescription pad for this pesky problem and Dr. Merrill Mitler of the Sleep Disorders Center, Scripps Clinic, La Jolla, California, says: "The most cost-effective way to treat insomnia is to give a patient a sleeping pill." Well, yes, and the most "cost-effective" way to treat tuberculosis is to let the patient die.

Insomnia is a widespread problem. About a third of all adults complain of at least occasional insomnia and it is a serious problem for many. It is very difficult to do meaningful testing on insomniacs because of the wide range of sleep required by different people. About one percent of the population only requires five hours of sleep a night, or even less. I wouldn't be able to turn on the stove or comb my hair with only five hours of sleep. At the other end of the sleep scale, some people need ten or more hours of sleep per night.

Some people who require only five hours sleep worry about not getting more. They are concerned about endangering their health by not getting enough rest. There is no evidence that they need worry. These people should learn to read more. One can get awfully smart with an extra three hours per day at the books. If you are getting only five hours of sleep a night and you need ten, then you definitely have a problem.

Action to Take

1. The best remedy for the serious insomniac is to take a short nap, an hour or less, in the early afternoon, i.e., no later than one o'clock. Most people, if they sleep any later in the afternoon, will compound their problem and have an even harder time sleeping that night.

2. If a patient is really desperate, I offer a compromise on sleeping pills — I am not nihilistic on drug therapy for insomnia. If you have gone two nights with-

out satisfactory sleep, I recommend a mild sleeper, such as valium, on the third night. This should not be repeated unless there are two more sleepless nights. I can't imagine a patient getting in trouble from sedatives on this type of schedule.

3. On the two sleepless nights, stop counting sheep and get up. Make some hot chocolate (seems to help) and read the journal, SLEEP, or the IRS manual on taxation. If those don't put you to sleep, you are incurable.

Ref: *International Herald Tribune*, August 27, 1992.

Before Cooking Fish, Give It a Hydrogen Peroxide Bath

The Consumers Union did a study of sanitary conditions and the state of the fish supply at markets around the U.S. What they found was far worse than a three-day-old dead fish and they raised a stink about it all the way to Washington.

From *Consumer Reports:* "Nearly half the fish we tested was contaminated by bacteria from human or animal feces ... for nearly 25 percent of our samples the bacteria count exceeded the upper limits of our test methods."

In all, half the fish was found to be rotten or "semi-rotten" and so unfit for human consumption. *Consumer Reports* added sardonically: "When bacteria counts hit ten million (colonies per gram) or more, fish should be headed for the grave rather than the dinner plate."

Perhaps rotten is too harsh an indictment here. Much of the bacteria is *surface* contamination and can be removed by wiping the surface of the fish carefully after rinsing in three percent hydrogen peroxide.

Ref: *Consumer Reports*, February 1992.

Chapter 6

Is Cancer Preventable?

I have a feeling that cancer is increasing at a frightening rate. People, not just in my practice, but personal friends and friends of friends, are dropping all around me. Do you have the same impression? Do you feel, as I do, that you are standing shoulder to shoulder with the "Son of the Morning Star," and the Indians are about to run you through?

We are told that in former pristine societies, such as Naureau, before bauxite mining brought them processed food and a life of indolence, people died a "natural death," i.e., they simply went to sleep at a hundred-and-something-or-other. This has also been reported in other hunter-gatherer societies in Africa and the Far East.

The only disease that's not preventable is death. But death is not really a disease, only the *end* of disease — the final solution to your problem. But shouldn't death be a simple stopping of the clock, a sleep from which you do not awake and not the result of some horrible disease? Isn't it possible that all the suffering we see, from what the insurance companies refer to as the "terminal illness," is brought on by how we lived? I don't mean that in a pejorative sense. After all, there are many things in our daily lives that we can't control, as I will briefly delineate below.

If cancer is not preventable, we are in deep trouble, because the "war on cancer," which Richard Nixon began 20 years ago, has been a failure comparable to Ouster's Last Stand. "Take no prisoners," Custer expostulated. He didn't and neither has Nixon, nor those taking up the cudgels since his initial declaration of war. The overall rate of cancer has *increased* since the inception of this great war, and the detection rate, in spite of all the propaganda about early detection curing cancer, has *decreased*. Our multi-billion-dollar cudgels against cancer have turned out to be nothing but wet noodles.

The incidence of cancer may, in fact, *be far worse* than we are told because autopsies are not as routinely done now as in the good old days. When I was in medical school, back when people listened to the radio at home and read books, you were graded on your ability to convince the next of kin to allow an autopsy. You would explain that it was for the good of science — and it really was. For once, we were telling the truth. We learn from our mistakes and we know the diagnosis of the deceased is wrong about half the time — but we don't know which half. The doctor got a lot of humility from autopsies. Unfortunately, lawyers also know about autopsies so a thousand years of good medical practice has been abandoned.

So if prevention is the answer to cancer, then why don't we prevent it? Is it the fault of the chemical companies, the fluoridators of your water, the cigarette companies, or even your doctor? The answer may be "all of the above" and many other factors not yet known, but we really don't know — and that's the problem.

We act like we know, but we really don't. Many so-called proofs are really suppositions. There is strong evidence that cigarette smoking, fluoride in your drinking water, and synthetic hormones cause cancer. But there is some doubt about even these suspects and the issue may be clouded by the need for a cofactor to be present before these agents are carcinogenic. For instance, synthetic hormones, such as those in birth control pills, may be more carcinogenic in the presence of cigarette smoke — and then they may not.

A fascinating example of cofactors being necessary to cause cancer is Burkitt's lymphoma, which is seen only in children in the tropics — especially equatorial Africa. The Epstein-Barr virus is clearly necessary in the development of Burkitt's cancer. But this cancer is found only where the population is also infected with malaria. When malaria is wiped out in a particular area, as it was in Uganda in the 1970s, Burkitt's lymphoma disappears. When malaria made a comeback in Uganda, so did Burkitt's lymphoma!

So here is a case where *two* cofactors are necessary for the development of a certain cancer: the E-B virus and the parasite, malaria. We have a lot to learn.

There are about 200 different cancers. They may all be the same but just look different because of the different cellular appearance of different tissues. I think they are all the same disease but their character varies with the tissue involved.

One aspect of cancer that would imply a strong environmental factor is the variance in the disease in different parts of the world as to frequency and the area of the body that it strikes. As examples, stomach cancer is 20 times more common in Japan than in Kuwait and breast cancer in Poland is five times less common than in San Francisco. It is these impressive statistics, all across the spectrum of cancer worldwide, that seem to shout to us that cancer is an environmental disease and so is indeed preventable.

But, as few causes of particular cancers are more than suspects, we don't know how to prevent them. We can't prevent something if we don't know for certain what causes it. And even if you are "fairly certain" of the cause, such as cigarette smoking causing lung cancer, how can it be prevented when one large group of the adult population doesn't take the danger seriously in spite of all the propaganda arrayed against it? Women, in particular, are guilty of this because they know that cigarette smoking tends to keep off weight and it's better to die slender than live fat. (Forgive me, Lord, for I have thinned.)

Action to Take

1. Don't get cancerphobia. Frequent checkups are dangerous to your health. Early detection has *not* been proven to prolong life or the quality of life and, in fact, aggressive treatments may shorten your life.

2. At the risk of boring you with repetition, avoid foods cooked in vegetable fats (which means all fast-food restaurants); avoid chlorinated/fluoridated water; get some sunshine every day and use full spectrum light at the work place and at home; don't smoke cigarettes; eat your spinach; and take plenty of garlic.

Ref: *New Scientist*, July 7, 1991.
     Acta Oncology 1989, 28, 5.

Risk of Cancer from Pesticides in Food

Every food you can possibly think of contains natural pesticides and carcinogens, even lettuce and that superstar of the health food stores, herbal tea. You want to be perfectly safe? Don't eat *anything*.

Because of this fact, Dr. Bruce Ames, professor of biochemistry at the University of California at Berkeley, and Lois S. Gold, director of the Carcinogenic Policy Project at the Lawrence Berkeley Laboratory, said that government cancer fears about traces of pesticide in food are vastly exaggerated. They also criticized the methods the government used in assessing carcinogens in foods. They asserted that the government focuses too heavily on rat studies, where the animals are given massive doses of the chemical being investigated (a dose the rats wouldn't face in ten lifetimes), and then, if the rats develop cancer, extrapolate the results to humans.

It's hard to call the results of these rat tests "science." If you stuff a goose with enough rich food, his liver will swell, creating an appetizer the French are particularly fond of. If you stuff a rat with enough of a particular chemical, whether it be water, salt, or aflatoxin, he's going to get sick. This chemical overdose weakens the immune system and allows cancer to develop without a fight. Obviously (at least I hope it's obvious), this proves nothing about the relationship of chemicals to cancer development in man. Roughly half of all known chemicals are carcinogenic at super-high levels of ingestion. According to Dr. Ames, the government's concentration on synthetic chemicals as carcinogens is "incredibly overblown."

Using the government's standard formula, Ames and Gold reported that the average cup of morning coffee may contain six to seven times the possible cancer hazard found in a liter of Silicon Valley's worst well-water tainted with trichloroethylene. Yet there is no evidence that coffee drinkers are dying in large numbers from drinking coffee. In 1980, I watched a TV interview with a 100-year-old lady. "To what do you attribute your long life?" the reporter asked. "I drinks ten cups of black coffee every day," she replied.

Ames and Gold also compared the results of government *pate' de foie gras* studies with their studies of the natural pesticides and natural carcinogenic agents found in foods. Their tests revealed that the American food basket is indeed teeming with potential carcinogens, but 99.9 percent of them are natural chemicals that foods develop as a self-defense against insects, or chemicals that develop as a byproduct of cooking. (I told you to eat raw meat.)

The researchers published their findings in *Science* magazine and a quote from their article brings the whole issue into focus: "Although the findings do not indicate that these *natural* dietary carcinogens are important to human cancer, they cast doubt on the relative importance for human cancer of the low-dose exposure to *synthetic* chemicals." (Emphasis added.)

If you want to worry about synthetic chemicals giving you cancer, why not concentrate on the obvious: the massive amounts of cancer-causing chlorine and fluoride that your local government puts into your drinking water. All the other chemicals combined, natural or synthetic, cannot compare with this gross contamination of your body.

Ref: *Science*, October 7, 1992.

Prostate Cancer — Leave It Alone

For years, we've been screaming at breast surgeons for unnecessarily mutilating too many women. But now we're finding that men aren't safe from the superfluous knife, either. Millions of men are getting unnecessary surgery for cancer of the prostate (that's *prostate*, not *prostrate* — you may be prostrate with prostate disease but you can't be prostrate from prostrate disease, unless you have a sleeping disorder.)

A recent study has confirmed what we have always suspected: There is "no clear benefit of choosing invasive therapy (surgery) in most cases" of prostate cancer, said the investigators in the *Journal of the American Medical Association*.

With the increase in sophistication of diagnostic methods, where we can almost determine how many angels can dance on the head of a pen, cancer is diagnosed extremely early. This has been heralded as an advance by the American Cancer Society and most doctors, but there have been two results of this early detection: (1) An apparent, but not real, increase in cures and (2) an increase in surgery. Notably absent from these results is an *actual* increase in the cure rate.

A small cancer in the prostate may, and usually will, stay within the confines of the gland for many years. Surgery in these slow-growing cancers is not only unnecessary, but is actually contraindicated and dangerous. Surgery can be fatal due to blood clots or infection.

So don't let your doctor frighten you into quick surgery. If you have cancer of the prostate, a few weeks of contemplation is not going to endanger your life. Get a second, or even a third, opinion. It's best to get the second opinion *out of town* — these doctors have to live together and so they don't want to offend their colleagues by saying a surgical procedure is unnecessary.

Ref: *Journal of the American Medical Association*^ May 26, 1993.

Chapter 7

Estrogen, Fat, and Cancer of the Breast

While you may have noticed by now that I have plenty of soap boxes when it comes to the modern practice of medicine, I also get much of my inspiration and direction from letters sent by my readers. In addition to offering valuable information, these letters also ask plenty of questions that broaden my research efforts and help keep me attuned to your interests.

We are told that the incidence of breast cancer is increasing at an alarming rate. Every article I read on the subject tells me that dietary fat is the cause. This propensity for researchers to pounce on diet for everything has me perplexed. Fat cannot be responsible for the *increase* in breast cancer. Most women my age (50) eat *less* fat than their mothers did. It must be something else. As you are the only doctor I know who has not fallen for the anti-animal fat propaganda, I would appreciate your opinion on this matter.

This is a tough question on a complex subject, but let's try to sort it out.

Mrs. Sprat ate plenty of fat — and probably outlived Jack. For years, women have been warned by the experts not to eat fat in order to avoid breast cancer.

We have maintained that this admonition was scientifically unwarranted and detrimental to good nutrition, as animal fat (but not all vegetable fats) is essential to good health.

Scientists at Brigham and Women's Hospital studied 90,000 women for eight years and concluded there was *no scientific evidence* for the assertion that a high-fat diet increased the incidence of breast cancer.

For more information on the Great Fat Fraud, see my book, *Eat Your Cholesterol.* You really don't have to eat like a Hindu to stay healthy, and yes, S.P., you can have your steak and eat it too.

Estrogen and Breast Cancer

S.P. asks several other questions which need to be answered here. She asks:

In the articles I have read on breast cancer, although they blame fat in the diet, there is always a veiled inference that estrogen is somehow to blame. But yet, we are told to take estrogen after menopause to avoid a heart attack! What is the best course of action in light of this conflicting advice?

Obviously, as S.P. alludes, you can't have it both ways. Should you take estrogen to avoid a heart attack and thus risk cancer or should you eschew estrogen to avoid cancer and thus risk a heart attack? This may look like the devil's choice, but let's look at it objectively. Most heart attacks are not fatal, while cancer of the breast is consistently fatal and is frequently slow and painful. The survival time with cancer is determined by the stage at which it is diagnosed — *today's treatments have not postponed the sounding of the final bell.* You may live longer after diagnosis, but that is because the diagnosis can be made earlier than in the past. You can worry about your illness longer, be made sick from chemotherapy earlier, and enrich the doctor more, but you can't live longer. So given the choice of taking estrogen to avoid heart attack (which probably doesn't work, anyway), or not taking estrogen to avoid cancer, which makes the most sense?

The estrogen fad is now being questioned and it's long overdue. Doctors still entertain the conceit that they can keep women young and disease-free until the day they drop by supplying them with artificial hormones. The drug industry, with the help of their ad agencies, has instilled this preposterous idea in the receptive heads of arrogant medicos who are long on pseudoscience and short on common sense concerning their role as guardians of the public health.

There have been very reliable reports on the association of exogenous estrogen therapy and cancer in general — not just breast cancer. Women taking estrogen also have a higher risk of uterine cancer. Even if they took the estrogen for only one or two years, *they remain at risk for cancer for at least ten years* after discontinuing the estrogen.

Meanwhile, most of the studies demonstrating a "protective effect" of estrogen against heart disease were financed by the drug industry and so are about as useful as rotten eggs.

Dr. Elizabeth Barrett-Connor from the University of California, San Diego, has now injected a dose of reality into this hormone business. The lower rate of coronary heart disease apparently associated with estrogen therapy, Dr. Barrett-Connor reports, is probably a result of better overall lifestyle. She points out that women not on estrogen therapy tend to be less educated, less health-conscious and are more likely to be heavy smokers.

Dr. Barrett-Connor's work was confirmed by a study at Northwestern University that showed *a 500 percent increase* in mortality from heart attacks among women who smoked.

Because of the grim facts about breast cancer therapy, I would avoid estrogen, including that in birth control pills (more on the pill in a minute). If you don't smoke cigarettes, you are not likely to have a heart attack.

Obesity a Factor?

S.P.'s next question: "Are fat women more likely to get breast cancer than thin women?"

Obesity gets blamed for everything — hypertension, diabetes, arteriosclerosis, premature death, gluttony, psychiatric disorders and world famine. None of it is true; some of it may be half true. No one really knows. (My answer is maybe — and that's final.)

But the American Cancer Society has come up with some statistics that are worth pondering, although I must admit I don't trust bureaucratic charity groups any more than I trust the news media. They report that men 40 percent overweight are more than twice as likely to die of cancer as those of normal weight. The pattern was only slightly less for women.

How About the Pill?

"Have any studies been done," S.P. asks "to see if there is a relationship between the number of years birth control pills have been taken and the incidence of breast cancer?"

The experts have been arguing for years as to whether the birth control pill, referred to as an OC (oral contraceptive), causes breast cancer. Most now agree that OCs do indeed cause breast cancer. A dramatic increase in the risk of breast cancer has occurred among premenopausal women who began using OCs before the age of 20, or who used OCs for more than five years before the age of 25. This was reported by a research team from Sweden at the University of Lund.

By contrast, women who started taking OCs *after* the age of 25, experienced "no substantial increase in the risk ... whatever their duration of OC use," said Dr. Hakan Olsson, who headed the study. "The results indicate the commencement of OC use *at an early age* is more important than the total duration of OC use for the risk of breast cancer."

A Bitter Pill

But susceptibility to breast cancer isn't the only thing you need to worry about with OCs. The pill can cause depression by altering tryptophan metabolism or, in a minority of cases, it can cause euphoria. Libido, the sexual drive, can be profoundly affected by birth control pills. This loss of sexual drive can cause further despair, which leads to even more depression of the sex urge.

The pill is an unnatural intrusion on the physiology of the female body. This intrusion can lead to many problems: cancer of the breast, cancer of the lung, cancer of the liver, pulmonary embolism (blood clot to the lung, sometimes fatal), acne, psychiatric and sexual changes, and probably other problems of which we are not yet aware.

Japanese: Pill or Kill?

S.P.'s last question: "Have Japanese women relied on birth control pills to the extent that North American women have, or are they more likely to use abortion for birth control?"

At present I can only answer part of this question. When I was in Japan in the late 1950s, the abortion rate was downright obscene (the procedure itself is obscene — you should watch one if you are "pro choice"). My impression is that the pill has now supplanted infanticide as the method of choice for birth control. If this is correct, then it would be interesting to know if there has been an increase in the incidence of breast cancer in the past 20 years. I'll check on it.

Ref: *Journal of the American Medical Association,* November 1992.
Time, November 2, 1992.
New England Journal of Medicine, 313, 969-972, 1985.
London Times, January 21, 1993.

Chapter 8

Vitamins in the Cure
of Cancer —
An Unprecedented Study

When I started practicing nutritional therapy in 1975, I never thought I would live to see the day when the National Cancer Institute (NCI) and a university would be conducting serious research into the prophylactic effect of vitamins on cancer. But serious researchers are now studying — with the sponsorship of the NCI, the Fred Hutchinson Cancer Research Center, and the University of Washington — the effect of vitamin A and beta carotene in the prevention of lung cancer. Beta carotene is similar to vitamin A, but does not have its toxic potential.

A diagnosis of lung cancer today offers a bleak future in that there is only a 15 percent survival rate at the end of five years and close to zero at the end of ten. Modern treatment is essentially worthless. But there is ample and growing evidence from animal studies to indicate that vitamin A and beta carotene may significantly reduce the risk of lung cancer. Although it is not known for certain, the anti-cancer effect is believed to be due to the "anti-oxidant" effect of the A vitamins. Just as iron rusts through oxidation (a chemical reaction with oxygen), so can cells. The "rust" in cells is the formation of harmful, oxidized chemicals that are thought to lead to the unrestrained cellular growth seen in cancer.

I don't like to see the government, in the guise of the NCI, involved in research on vitamins, a field in which they have a powerful negative bias. But the feds have so distorted medical research in this country, through monopoly of funds and oppressive regulations, that there is no other choice but to go along and hope it's not an ambush. It very well could be a "cooked up" experiment to discredit preventive vitamin therapy. I hope I'm wrong!

Ref: *Seattle Post Intelligencer* via the *Townsend Letter.*

Folic Acid — It's About Time

The word is out: "Folic acid ... has suddenly been thrust into the nutritional limelight."

It may have been suddenly thrust into the limelight, but many of us in the natural medicine field have been using large doses of folic acid *for 20 years.*

I first got excited about folic acid (which is also called folate or folacin) from reading the pioneer work of Harvard's Dr. Hardin Jones concerning the importance of vitamin B_6 in the prevention of arteriosclerosis. His research led me to folic acid and its importance in the same metabolic syndrome. Jones discovered that if meat is overcooked, vitamin B_6 is destroyed or inactivated, resulting in a serious metabolic problem and consequent arteriosclerosis; the same thing happens with the destruction of folic acid.

The problem has to do with an amino acid called homocysteine which is a break-down product of meat protein. If the meat has been overcooked, resulting in a temporary deficiency in folate and vitamin B_6, then the homocysteine, *which is highly conducive to hardening of the arteries* ("atherogenic"), will not be converted to another amino acid, called cystathionine, which is not atherogenic. So for 20 years I, and many other "radicals" in the medical profession, have been recommending 100 mg per day of vitamin B6, especially if the patient eats large amounts of overcooked meat, and a minimum of 1000 micrograms of folic acid.

The trouble is, you don't get credit for the heart attacks you have prevented because you can't see what didn't happen. It's much more heroic to save someone from dying of a heart attack, as the result is obvious — you can charge more, too. And that's why prevention-oriented doctors never get rich. Most people just don't have the imagination, or self-control, to understand or benefit from preventive medicine.

In my research, I found an interesting study that indicates a cancer connection with a lack of folic acid. In some experimental animals, folate deficiency doubles the rate of colon cancer. Cancers of the cervix, lung, esophagus, and breast have been associated with a low blood level of folic acid — and we are not talking about extremely low levels, either — prompting some researchers to suggest that the minimum daily requirement of folacin should be raised. So what does the Food and Nutrition Board of the National Research Council do to protect your health? *They cut the recommended daily allowance in half for men and less than half for women.* Some nutrition experts had the courage to call this action "a grave misjudgment."

My next encounter with the remarkable benefits of folacin was from reading the reports of Dr. Kurt Oster on the use of this vitamin in the prevention of hardening of the arteries secondary to the drinking of homogenized milk. The homogenization process breaks up the fat globules in milk, making them small enough to pass through the bowel wall. The fat has on its surface an enzyme called xanthine oxidase which does not enter the circulation when attached to the larger, natural fat globules. Xanthine oxidase is known to be highly atherogenic and will turn the arteries of experimental animals into concrete pipes.

Folic acid will protect the arteries from the destructive effects of xanthine oxidase. If you drink homogenized milk, you should take a minimum of 1000 micrograms of folic acid daily. I am not suggesting that you drink homogenized milk or any of the other fractionated abominations — skim, two percent, etc. — that are passed off as milk.

Action to Take

1. Don't be impressed by these organizations that tell you how to take nutrients. They are (a) often politically motivated, (b) usually ill-informed on the latest nutritional research, as it usually doesn't appear in the establishment journals (until years later - folic acid is an excellent example of "prestigious advisory groups" running off in the wrong direction), and (c) they are afraid of each other and don't want to recommend something that is not within the majority thinking; it's called "science by vote."

2. Eat or drink foods rich in folic acid such as fresh orange juice (*not* concentrate), medium-rare chicken or beef liver, lentils, and cereals.

3. Take 1000 micrograms of folic acid daily in tablet form. Although it has become uncommon, folate can mask pernicious anemia, caused by a deficiency of B_{12}, so have your B_{12} level checked.

Chapter 9

Chelation Works!

Chelation therapy, the treatment of hardening of the arteries with a synthetic amino acid administered into a vein, has been almost ignored to death by conventional medicine. If it were to be accepted as a valid modality, which it is, the pharmaceutical industry, the doctor industry, and the surgical industry would suffer grievous harm.

Why the insurance companies would be opposed to a therapy that prolongs life is beyond me. Chelation therapy, by prolonging health, and perhaps life, causes *a positive cashflow* to the insurance companies — the longer you live, the longer you pay premiums and defer their cost of "insuring" your life. Why would they refuse to pay for a treatment that increases profits? The only answer I can come up with is the don't-rock-the-boat syndrome: We're making money — don't change anything.

Ignoring this rapidly growing technology didn't work, so then the horror stories began to appear in the lay and scientific press: Chelation can destroy the kidneys (true if misused); Chelation can dissolve your bones causing osteoporosis (not true — it may even *help* osteoporosis); It doesn't work (haven't heard that one recently because it obviously does work).

But the most effective and invidious ploy against chelation has not been dark conspiracies, but simply the blaming of terminal patients* deaths on the treatment. Here's a typical scenario: A 70-year-old man has had two "bye-pass" operations. He is in such bad shape that he can't go to the bathroom without help. His brain is obtunded and he is considering suicide. He has a chronic bladder infection and possibly an infection of a heart valve secondary to the operation. He had a stroke follow- ing surgery — not an uncommon occurrence — and can- not use his right hand. And certainly not least important, he is in constant pain from the huge incision the sur- geons had to make through his chest in order to stomp on his heart.

The family, realizing that he is worse off than before the surgery, takes him to a doctor specializing in chela- tion therapy. They are not stupid suckers; they are not uneducated peasants; the facts are quite simple: Dad went in for coronary by-pass surgery; they spent $100,000 of the insurance company's and their own money; Dad's much worse off. It's as simple as that. Modern medicine has made an invalid out of a loving husband, father, and grandfather.

According to modern medicine, it's time to give up. I forget who said it: "It's better to die than go against the faculty of medicine." But people are now turning against the "faculty of medicine" and are seeking other avenues of therapy — in droves. And chelation is an alternative to drugs and surgery that has been rapidly gaining the con- fidence of people the world over.

If you just want the cold, hard facts on chelation therapy, then move on to page 35. But you should read this story. Medicine isn't just chemicals — it's about *peo- ple*, good and bad.

The Human Side

As with so many things in life, I became a chelation advocate (and Public Enemy Number One with my medical society) because of a chance encounter with a dying man in an emergency facility at a small hospital in Port Charlotte, Florida. One of my colleagues had asked me to switch nights on duty with her, which I did. At eight o'clock in the evening, a 45-year-old man was brought in with severe chest pain. As I was interviewing him, he had a seizure. We were well-trained in cardiac emergencies — this was Retirementville, U.S.A., where many people died a cardiac death every day — we really knew our stuff, and were proud of it. Chest pain plus convulsion equals ventricular fibrillation — and a rapid death unless immediate action is taken.

My patient, whose name was Al, had chosen the perfect place to have a massive heart attack. Because of his complaint, we had immediately started an intravenous drip when he came in "just in case." The electrodes had been placed on his chest in the ambulance so we had immediate confirmation of the diagnosis when he convulsed: ventricular fibrillation. The electrical paddles, used to convert the heart to a normal rhythm, were at my side, a breathing tube was ready, and the oxygen was flowing. Everything required to bring Al back from the brink of death was in place and immediately applied. The whole life-saving procedure — defibrillation, intubation, respiration, the administering of certain drugs — took four of us about 45 seconds. Boy, was he lucky to be at the right place at the right time.

His wife witnessed this entire drama and, after he recovered, told him about it. He was one of the few patients who ever thanked me for saving his life. Most of them never knew who yanked them from the jaws of death; they only knew the doctors they met after regaining consciousness in their hospital bed the following day — those doctors got the credit and the Christmas cards; we got the complaints about the bill: "What's this for — I've never seen *you!*"

Tabloid Wisdom

A month later, Al brought a tabloid newspaper, the *National Enquirer*, into the emergency department and asked me about a "new treatment" called chelation therapy, prominently featured in the tabloid. He was considering taking this miracle therapy. It was said to "dissolve away" the rust and crud in the arteries and thus enable the patient to avoid coronary by-pass surgery. He had had one of those, and one was enough.

I patiently explained to Al, an uneducated, very smart, and street-wise Italian restauranteur who could afford any treatment he wished, and who wanted to stay viable for his pretty new bride, Marty, that this was a *tabloid* article and therefore wasn't worth the yellow paper it was written on.

As I said, Al was street-wise; I wasn't: "Listen, Doc, just because this ain't in the AMA whata-you-call-it journal don't mean it's a lie. I know it ain't the truth, necessarily, but do *you* know enough about it to say it's bull—?" He really had me. It was difficult for him to talk to me like that, he told me later after we had become good friends. He had an immense respect for doctors but he'd jump on anything, or anybody, where his health was concerned — Al was a survivor.

After a number of false starts, I found, to my surprise, an organization of doctors who advocated chelation therapy. I studied their research information, listened to their case histories, went to their meetings, and have been an enthusiastic supporter and practitioner of chelation therapy ever since. I have treated hundreds of patients, starting with Al, and have seen some truly remarkable results.

The story of Al has a sad, and for me, frustrating ending. He did so well on chelation that he began to feel invulnerable — so much so that he went back to smoking and working 14 hours a day. In spite of this abuse of himself, he continued his lifestyle completely free of pain or other symptoms of heart disease for five years. He felt so great that he decided to stop the treatments in spite of Marty's urging and my warnings.

Six months after stopping the treatments he had a massive heart attack and died in the same hospital where we met. *The doctors blamed the chelation therapy and me for his death.* Matty's retort to them was even more unprintable than Al's would have been. She could have cooperated with these doctors, ruined my career and made a bundle — "pretty young girl's husband dies at the hand of a quack" — the local medical society said so — case closed; it would have been easy. I tell you this story so you can appreciate how tough it is for a doctor to practice outside the mainstream. I'm surprised we aren't *all* in jail.

The Scientific Side

If you're picking up the chelation story here, then you've missed the reason why you should have great respect and admiration for your chelation doctor, but you probably do anyway.

Chelation refers to the ability of certain chemicals to bind with calcium, iron, and other metals, and remove them from the body. We know there is a lot of calcium in those plaques that appear in the arteries of patients with "arteriosclerosis." Presumably, if calcium could be "clawed out" of a constricted vessel ("chelation" comes from the Greek word, *chele*, meaning claw) then the plaque could be slowly dissolved away. This is probably *part* of the explanation for how chelation works, but there is a lot more to it than that. In fact, the more we learn, the more mysterious it gets.

The primary chelating agent used in clinical practice is called EDTA, ethylene diamine tetraacetic acid. EDTA is a synthetic amino acid first produced in Germany in 1930. It was used as a preservative in cloth, and later as a stabilizer for food, such as Mayonnaise (check your Hellman's Mayonnaise label and you'll see that you have been eating EDTA all your life). In the 1950s, Dr. Norman E. Clarke, chairman of the research department, Providence Hospital, Detroit, Michigan, began research on the effects of EDTA chelation therapy on cardiovascular disease.

"I've Seen Only Benefits"

Dr. Clarke's motivation for investigating the possibility that EDTA would do in the human body what it did for mayonnaise, a rather preposterous idea on the face of it, was based on the hopelessness he felt after 30 years of treating arteriosclerotic heart disease with no positive results: "I knew, having been in cardiology quite a number of years, that arteriosclerotic vascular disease was a helpless, hopeless situation for the cardiologist." Few cardiologists, then or now, have the courage to admit they do very little to help their patients.

Dr. Clarke gave some historic testimony before the Scientific Board of the California Medical Society in 1976 that few doctors are aware of. He reported that he had personally administered 120,000 infusions of EDTA chelation and never saw "any serious toxicity whatsoever. I've seen only benefits."

The first dramatic results seen by Dr. Clarke were in patients with blocked arteries as a result of diabetic vascular disease. He reported cases of gangrene of the toes, due to blockage of the arteries, that were saved from amputation of the foot by intravenous chelation therapy. This dramatic reversal of a "surgical problem" by the use of a medication had never been achieved before. Surgeons were not enthusiastic, however, and, strangely, neither were most cardiologists. Almost 20 years after Dr. Clarke's remarkable testimony, they're *still* not enthusiastic.

He next reported on the use of chelation in elderly patients with senility due to arterial blockage in the brain. He had similar dramatic results and remarked to the scientific board: "After all these years and after all that experience, I am just as certain as can be that EDTA chelation therapy is the best treatment that has ever been brought out for occlusive vascular disease."

I would like to emphasize that Dr. Clarke was not reporting on Alzheimer's disease, another matter entirely, involving a younger population. Alzheimer's generally affects people in their late 50s and early 60s, who lose their minds as though they were much older. It's basically an early senility, often accompanied with frank psychosis and eventual violence — a terrible fate, and one in which chelation therapy has been, in most cases, disappointing. Because of the ability of chelation to bind and eliminate toxic metals from the body, the therapy *might* be useful as a preventive, but there is no way to prove that.

The Cancer Connection

Whether or not it helps Alzheimer's, though, one solid reason for preventive chelation therapy is this: *there is compelling evidence that chelation can prevent cancer.*

In 1972, a Swiss report indicated a preventive effect against cancer as a result of chelation therapy. The research had been done on the use of chelation in the treatment of lead poisoning but the follow up studies on those treated revealed that the participants in the lead treatment study had a 600 percent decrease in the incidence of cancer as compared to people in the same community not given chelation.

It is not generally known, even by most doctors, that almost all chemotherapy procedures used in the treatment of cancer involve some form of chelation. Most antibiotics work through chelation and even aspirin is a chelating agent. So if your doctor says he doesn't believe chelation is valid therapy, tell him he doesn't know what he is doing, from the biochemical point of view, and to go back to his chemistry books. (Be sure to have another doctor lined up first.)

The one area where chelation is accepted is in the treatment of heavy metal poisoning — especially lead. They can't deny it works there. But it is also effective in the removal of iron, a far more serious problem in the general population than lead poisoning.

Americans in general are overloaded with iron, primarily due to a misguided food industry that adds iron to foods as a "fortification," because the experts at the PDA say its good for us. Well, it isn't good for *most* of us — it's *bad* for us. Excessive iron leads to hardening of the arteries and iron is probably the most important toxin in our foods — not cholesterol, not fat, not salt — *iron.*

Other Benefits

Patients who come in for chelation for their vascular disease are often pleasantly surprised to note their arthritis improved. The reason for this is not known. It may be due to removal of iron, or calcium, or both, or it may be due to the improvement of the circulation to the joint —

or all, or none, of the above. But, for whatever reason, the improvement in arthritis is often dramatic.

In my experience, the first sign of improvement is often seen in the skin. Many patients remark on the improvement in their skin color, the disappearance of blemishes and better skin turgor.

With heart patients, the first sign of improvement is usually an increase in exercise tolerance. I have had patients who had difficulty crossing the living room who, after 20 treatments, could walk to the mail box, a hundred yards down the path, with no difficulty. (Sometimes my bill would be in there. It's easier to collect when the patient can walk to the mail box and he couldn't before.)

The procedure is relatively simple. The doctor will check you out for kidney malfunction, heart failure, and any other condition that would indicate the need for a modified, more cautious approach. There are few patients who cannot tolerate the treatment. You will sit in a reclining chair for two to three hours taking an intravenous drip. The most common side effect is boredom, so bring an interesting book.

You should commit yourself to 30 treatments. Don't expect miracles with the first infusion — you didn't get in this terrible shape overnight.

There are other methods of clearing the arteries which are complementary to chelation. Hydrogen peroxide, also given intravenously, has a chelating effect, although the mechanism by which it works is different. And we now have a third therapeutic weapon, photoluminescence, which treats the blood with light and has a mechanism of action similar to hydrogen peroxide — a marked increase in the oxygenation of the body's organs and tissues. In the chelation protocol of the near future, all three of these treatment modalities will be used together for the alleviation of many diseases.

Action to Take

1. Read Dr. Morton Walker's book on this subject, *The Chelation Answer.*

2. Watch your iron intake — read my articles to see if you should, or should not, be taking iron.

3. Find a doctor who understands the importance of iron metabolism and ask him to check your ferritin level (a mirror of your iron status). If he says he'll just do a serum iron level then he doesn't understand the problem.

4. If you are over 60, or unhealthy at any age, take preventive chelation therapy. Listed below are organizations that can help you to find a qualified therapist.

American College for the Advancement of Medicine
Box 3427
Laguna Hills, CA 92654
Phone: In CA, 714-583-7666; Outside CA, 800-532-3688.
Send a SASE with $0.55 postage for free list.

International Bio-Oxidative Medicine Foundation
P.O. Box 891954
Oklahoma City, OK 73113
Phone: 405-478-4266
Send written request and $5.00 for doctor list.

American Board of Chelation Therapy
70 West Huron
Chicago, IL 60610
Phone: 800-356-2228
Call or write (send SASE) for free list.

Chapter 10

Salt of the Earth

Did you know that the natives in the Himalayas often live to be 100 years old, or more? The American Heart Association says that the long life span of these natives is due to apricot pits, but it isn't. There's nothing wrong with apricot pits — I put my cancer patients on them when we can find them.

Anthropologists from Case Western Reserve University in Cleveland, Ohio reported their findings on blood pressure in Tibet at a National Academy of Sciences Symposium in Washington, D.C. several years ago. Their report indicated that the diet of the Phala nomads would be considered close to original sin by American experts - milk, butter, cheese, sheep, antelope, yak, a considerable amount of salt, and practically no fruits or vegetables. But their blood pressure averages are far lower than in the U.S. This evidence has been completely ignored.

In the United States, salt gets almost as much flak as that other essential nutrient, cholesterol. As with cholesterol reduction, most doctors who recommend a low intake of salt for their hypertension patients or, in general "to prevent high blood pressure," haven't done their homework. And of course the food companies like the false propaganda against salt because it stimulates the sale of salt substitutes, which sell at a much higher price than regular salt.

"Refining" the World's Health

The Industrial Revolution, often blamed for all of man's problems, relieved man of much of the manual drudgery that had kept him chained to the soil. It has brought him marvels of transportation, surgery, and communications that were inconceivable as recently as 1900. But there has been a downside — the advent of mind-numbing reactionary socialist propaganda, monopolistic corporations and governments, Roseanne Barr (the death of taste) — and the refining process. The refining of salt, although not generally recognized, is one of the reasons for the breakdown of health in societies all over the world.

In order to give salt a fair shake, let's look at some important basic facts: (1) No studies have ever proven that salt causes hypertension (high blood pressure) and (2) severe salt restriction may actually *cause* hypertension.

In spite of these findings in favor of an adequate salt intake, the Surgeon General, the Department of Health and Human Services, and that professional organization that always seems to come up on the wrong side of health and nutrition issues, the American Heart Association, all recommend curtailing salt intake.

People spend a lot of money on mineral supplements that could be obtained naturally and cheaply - simply by buying the right kind of salt. Note that I said the right kind of salt. I am referring, as you might have guessed, to sea salt. But it's not as simple as that (like most things). People talk about fat as if all fat was the same thing. They talk the same way about water, milk, light, vitamins, and "sea salt" as if they all sprang from nature and were unsullied by man.

Salt, next to light, is probably our most neglected and misunderstood nutrient. Even the health food folks, for the most part, don't realize that the salt they sell as "natural sea salt" isn't natural at all. Any salt, if you go back far enough, is from the sea, but if that was 5,000 years ago it no longer counts as sea salt. So, theoretically, even Morton's is "natural sea salt."

It doesn't take a geologist to determine whether a salt offered for sale is legitimate natural sea salt. The real thing will have the following characteristics:

1. It is light grey in color and, on standing, the color darkens slightly at the base of the container.

2. It is moist to the touch and remains moist even when kept in cool storage for long periods of time.

3. It is formed of small, precisely cubic, crystals (look at a few grains under magnification).

The magnesium salts are responsible for the moistness of natural salt. If the magnesium has been refined out, the salt will "pour when it rains." When natural salt stands, the moisture will settle to the bottom of the container. So the salt should be mixed every few days in order to keep it "alive." The light grey color is caused by the dozens of minerals present in natural salt.

The French "natural sea salt" is a good example as to how the nutrient-seeking public a being misled into using falsely labeled products bought at great expense. French "natural sea salt" is a thoroughly refined product, as sparkling white as refined sugar and is nutrient-free — just like the M&Ms from the movie refreshment counter. French "natural sea salt" is bulldozed up from the shores of the highly polluted Mediterranean. If they didn't refine it, you would succumb from the toxins.

Mexican salt is another example of mislabeling and false advertising. But this time it's the Japanese who are being fed an inferior product — before they ship it back to the U.S. for sale in soy sauce and other "natural" Japanese products. Salt is a state monopoly in Japan so, naturally, things are a little mucked up. Some Japanese companies are getting around the bureaucrats by adding back the minerals taken out in the refining process. This salt is *still* not as good as clean, unrefined, hand-harvested natural sea salt.

No supplementation can equal the wealth of minerals, in the right balance, found in natural sea salt. In the industrial refining of salt, as many as 82 trace minerals and essential micronutrients are removed, leaving nothing but industrial grade sodium chloride. For many of these micronutrients, salt is the only readily available source. "Parts is parts" as they used to say in the chicken commercial, but there are salts and there is sodium chloride, the chemical, which is probably what you are using at the dinner table.

The Body Does What the Alchemists Couldn't — Change Lead to Gold

Well, it might change lead to gold if it had a mind to, but there is no doubt that the body does change, by "transmutation," sodium into vital potassium. Because of this ability, natural sea salt and your body work a bio-electronic miracle.

Also, natural sea salt is an alkalinizer. An acidity of the body fluids is believed to be the cause of, or a contributor to, many illnesses. In severe trauma and infections, the body needs an emergency supply of potassium to repair the imbalance. The easiest way to provide this is to administer by mouth small doses of light grey Celtic sea salt dissolved in distilled water. A level teaspoonful in an eight-ounce glass of distilled water is enough. Taking this solution once a day for a maximum of four days can often work wonders. The potassium will be replenished quickly as the body "transmutes" the sodium into potassium.

People are often surprised at the dramatic improvement in health seen with this treatment. The acid/base level is quickly restored, allergies and skin conditions clear up, and there is a higher resistance to infections. This self-treatment is perfectly safe unless you have severe kidney disease, a pituitary abnormality, or salt-sensitive hypertension (most hypertension is *not* salt-sensitive, as we will explain below).

The Four Body Fluids — Internal Oceans

There are four "internal oceans" of the body that require constant and frequent replenishment of vital minerals, many of which are unavailable from foods -even though they may be present in some foods. That is why unrefined, unadulterated, naturally harvested sea salt is essential to prevent premature aging and the warding off of many diseases. The four internal oceans are:

1. *The plasma, or noncellular portion of the blood.* The white cells, the red cells, the platelets, and other solid elements (including fats and proteins) float along in this internal stream in your veins, arteries, and capillaries.

2. *The extracellular fluid.* This is the "juice" that bathes all your cells and tissues.

3. *The lymphatic circulatory system.* This is a system of tiny vessels that collects the "juices" around your cells and puts them back into the veins for reprocessing and replenishment of minerals and other nutrients, such as oxygen. So these juices are processed back into blood plasma.

4. *The cerebrospinal fluid.* This is the fluid that bathes your brain and spinal cord.

All of these "internal oceans," remarkably similar to sea water, are interconnected and each can affect the other.

The human fetus spends the first nine months of its life floating in a slightly modified ocean, called amniotic fluid, almost identical to those mentioned above. From the moment of conception to death we are dependent on these internal seas, and these internal seas are dependent on sea salt for maximum health and a long life. If any of the trace elements found in unrefined sea salt are lacking, the body will be denied essential bioelectric forces and enzymatic actions that are necessary for maximum function and efficiency of the body.

Better Restrict Your Salt Intake — The Doctor Said So

As we mentioned earlier, doctors talk about salt as if all salts were the same — salt is salt. This simply reveals their ignorance on the subject and the irony of this is that *they are right in condemning commercial, refined salt, but for the wrong reasons.* What good does it do to condemn something if your condemnation endangers the health of the patient because you didn't replace the unhealthy product with one that will *help* the patient?

Refined salt, such as Morton's, is as devoid of natural vitamins and minerals as white bread. The reason it pours is because it contains ferrocyanide, yellow prussiate of soda, tricalcium phosphate, alumino-calcium silicate, and sodium alumino-silicate. Silicates, as you probably know, are basically sand. All of these additives are anti-caking agents used to prevent the salt from mixing with water and thus causing "caking." But if the salt won't mix with water, it won't mix with the sea water in your body and is therefore useless and is an anti-nutrient.

The reason for this stripping of the nutrients from salt is twofold. The primary reason is that the salt on your table was not manufactured for you. It was manufactured for the chemical, plastic, metallurgical, and atomic industries. It is simply an *industrial chemical* passed off on you as a food. The other incentive to extract the minerals from natural salt is so that they can be sold back to you and industry at a healthy markup.

There is no retail store, "health food," "macrobiotic," or otherwise, that sells "natural sea salt." The so-called natural salts, such as Lima, Si-Salt, and Muramoto, have been machine-harvested and either washed, boiled, skimmed, or oven-dried.

Industrial Grade Salt

Refined salt, such as Morton's, is almost completely devoid of natural vitamins and minerals. These important nutrients were stripped from salt for industrial purposes, with little thought being given to the effect this process would have on your body.

If the Food Chemical Codex — a federal regulatory agency that sets standards for the composition and manufacturing of foods — were doing its job properly, it would outlaw the salt on your dinner table. Apparently, the Codex chemists and biologists are unaware of the difference between commercial salt and unrefined sea salt.

Instead of going to knowledgeable biochemists who would be unprejudiced in their evaluation of the nutrient value and safety of various salts, the government Codex regulators went to the industrial salt-makers and asked *them* to define safe, nutritious, edible salt. Ninety-three percent of industrial salt production goes to industry. The manufacturer's standard procedure is to extract all those pesky "contaminants" (such as magnesium and potassium) that can be sold at an immense profit to industry, including the nutrition industry. So when Codex came knocking, the salt miners had a ready answer: Our "pure" salt is just right for humans and "must not contain over 2 1/2 percent of trace minerals." So the criterion for "pure" edible salt became the extraction of most of the essential nutrients, thus changing one of nature's most perfectly balanced foods into a harmful chemical.

To fatten their sweetheart deal, the chemical salt-makers wrote into the regulations that their industrial salt, which was about to be transformed into a "pure food," could contain up to two percent of chemical additives, such as bleaches, anti-caking agents (sand), and conditioners. The industrial salt producers had to have these two regulations — stripping salt of all its nutrients along with the impurities and the adding back of chemicals — tailored to their liking, because they knew they could not develop a whole-food salt without giving up the minerals that they sold *back* to the health food industry at immense profit.

Some health food stores will sell U.S. crude salt, the implication being that it is comparable to crude, unrefined sugar. *Nothing could be further from the truth. Unrefined industrial salt should never* be used as a food, as their sources are heavily contaminated with toxic heavy metals, concrete efflorescence, and other pollutants. Even if this salt is handpicked in order to get out the darker, obviously contaminated crystals, much of the contaminants are locked within the crystals.

Is Restricting Salt in the Diet Bad Medicine?

Conventional scientific wisdom has said that there are few salt-related health problems from *too little* salt; only *too much* salt in the diet presents a problem. But again the "parts is parts" confusion: Most people in the world (and it is a worldwide problem) get too much stripped, contaminated salt and *none* of the health-giving, pure sea salt. The current medical mantra, "Our body can function on no added salt at all, or on a severely restricted salt intake," is simply bad medical advice. Clean, unrefined sea salt should be considered an *essential nutrient* complex, a food enjoyed by not one person in a thousand in the industrial world, a food that is condemned by 99 percent of the medical profession!

To understand the importance of natural sea salt, one must understand the health importance of sodium. Most medical biologists and physicians think of sodium alone, as they would arsenic or lead, and not in relation to other essential elements such as water and potassium. *Sodium is key to a healthy life* as it works in close chemical cooperation with chlorine, potassium, calcium, and other ions.

Sodium, in the form of sodium chloride (salt), plays an essential role in digestion, starting from the moment food enters your mouth. Salt, and thus sodium, activates the primary digestive enzyme in the mouth, salivary amylase. Sodium activates the taste buds whereas the "salt substitute," containing a mixture of sodium chloride and potassium chloride, does so only weakly, depending on how much *real* salt (sodium chloride), is in the product. That's why "salt substitutes" are not as satisfying as the real thing and people often add more of the substitute in order to get more of the real salt.

Further down the digestive tract, in the stomach, sodium continues its good work. Sodium chloride generates hydrochloric acid in the parietal cells of the stomach wall, an essential secretion for proper digestion (and *not* the bad guy inappropriately blamed for peptic ulcers, which are caused by a bacterium, *helicobacter pylori*).

The excess of potassium, in relation to sodium, in fake salts can cause great harm to your health. Enzymatic pathways are blocked by the abnormal sodium-potassium ratio and so the production of hydrochloric acid is blocked. Most diets, *especially vegetarian diets*, require added salt to maintain the sodium-potassium ratio. With the presence of salt, the partially digested food is high in acidity and thus the stomach can produce sodium bicarbonate which is essential to digestion and proper acid/base balance in the body. *Without salt, no digestion is possible.*

Vegetarians and Salt

If you are a vegetarian, I must have gotten your attention with that last paragraph. Vegetarians have been led to believe that their veggies supply all the salt they need in their diet. This is completely false. Why are salt blocks provided for grazing animals? They are provided with this salt source because every farmer knows that without it, his vegetarian animals will get sick. Herbivorous animals do two things: eat and sleep. When awake, they eat, but they can't eat enough grass or hay to supply their salt needs — *and neither can a grazing human.*

In fact, the situation is even worse for humans trying to imitate the eating habits of cows and horses, because domesticated grains and vegetables contain even lower amounts of salt. A pure vegetarian has to eat almost constantly and imbibe quarts of juices to get enough salt. Actually, fruits and vegetables are nearly salt-free. That is why vegetarians have a craving for salty junk foods or, for that matter, salt in any way they can get it. Salt is the single element required for the proper breakdown of plant carbohydrates into usable and assimilable human food. A salt-free, vegetarian diet is a sure ticket to the hospital and a premature old age.

Vegetarians are also prone to sugar addiction. The physiological explanation for this: Glucosides in grains are not digested without the presence of salt. As the body is denied these natural sugars, a deficiency develops and there is an insatiable desire to eat sweets.

High Blood Pressure and Salt

Only a third of hypertensive patients are "salt-sensitive" and therefore need to have their salt intake restricted. These patients have a low level of the kidney hormone, renin. The other two thirds of the hypertensive population also have a hormonal problem, but it is unrelated to their dietary salt and more harm than good will result from restricting their salt intake.

This majority of hypertensives has a *high* renin level rather than a low one and their body salt is already excessively reduced. Putting these patients on a restricted salt diet may lead to an even higher blood pressure, salt starvation, and possible disaster. We are indebted to John H. Laragh, M.D., at the Hypertension Center, New York-Cornell Medical Center, for his landmark work on hypertension and salt.

The Magnesium Problem

While fake salt can lead to an excess of potassium, as we have described, refined salt (which is also fake salt) can lead to a deficiency in the vital mineral magnesium. Refined salt contains only 0.03 percent or, in some cases, 0.00 percent, of magnesium instead of the 0.7 percent found in natural sea salt. Magnesium is absolutely vital to health and life itself. Magnesium deficiency leads to heart disease, abnormal bone metabolism, and other deficiencies in the blood.

Magnesium deficiency is prone to develop in the elderly and is related to impotency and senility. Because of magnesium-deficient soils and the eating of magnesium-deficient junk food, unrefined sea salt is absolutely essential to prevent premature aging.

Pure Salt from France

Fortunately for us, a well-qualified scientist, Dr. Jacques de Langre, has evaluated the salts of the world and has found the near-perfect salt in France:

"Cold, active, northern seas, because of upwelling and other marine and climactic conditions, offer the advantages of a rich mix of minerals.... Winds not only dry more than sun alone, but 'load' the salt flats and stacks with additional trace elements, mainly iodine salts. These additional nutrients are carried as spray from the crests of waves....

"The method used for gathering salt from natural flats and effectively separating it from the hard soil is crucial to the production of health-giving salt. There must be some constant eddying movement in the brine — a kinetic crystallization — over and through the clay flats.... In order to ionize and harmonize the trace elements by the clay's filtering action, the final hand-raking of the moist crystals is done by artisans with such a skillful, light touch that almost no particles of clay appear in the finished natural product.

"In the case of Flower of the Ocean' salt, an almost white Celtic salt which is harvested traditionally and is rare because it crystallizes naturally on top of the water only during the hottest days of the harvest, it contains no clay particles at all and yields tiny white crystals. The gathering is done delicately from the top layer of the brine and thus no clay is ever trapped in the final, smaller crystal structure.

"Both methods just described are still followed by a dedicated group of professional natural salt farmers in Europe who perpetuate the traditional skills passed down through generations from antiquity. When harvested in these ways, both of these natural sea salts are highly beneficial to anyone's health as they possess therapeutic qualities that are capable to restore balance, even in long-standing chronic afflictions."

But be warned: not all salt from France is this nutritious sea salt. Many French products labeled as "natural sea salt" are being aggressively marketed through gourmet shops and health food stores. These are totally refined, glistening white sea salt that has been extracted by industrial bulldozers from concrete beds at the Mediterranean coast line, which is more polluted than San Francisco Bay.

Dr. de Langre has found only one French sea salt, which is one of the few sea salts in the world, that has the full compliment of minerals and is completely free of toxins and other contaminants. That salt is the one described above from the coast of Brittany. There are other equally pure and mineralized salts in the world but they are few in number.

Where Can You Get Real Salt?

I never like recommending only one product as it connotes self-aggrandizement and conflict of interest — you know, a Whitewater type of thing. But if there is really only one product that fills the bill, then I am going to recommend it. It goes without saying — well maybe it doesn't go without saying — that I have no financial interest in the Grain and Salt Society of Magalia, California. I must confess that I have received free salt from them on occasion, but what are you going to do if they refuse to cash your checks — do without? They really are grateful for our endorsement and I hope they get rich. They're the kind of folks who will use the money for a good purpose. There is more than a grain of salt in this report and I hope you will act upon it for the better health of your family. Here's how to get started: The Grain and Salt Society, P.O. Box DD, Magalia, CA 95954, Tel: 916-873-0294, Fax: 916-872-5524.

The Grain and Salt Society has three sample packages that range in price from $16.40 to $36.40. I recommend that you try the more expensive package. It includes a 1/2 pound of each of their salts and a book explaining the difference between the three. For more information, please call these nice folks and ask them all about their products — and don't forget to ask about their membership prices.

Chapter 11

Hey, Doc! What About...?

Every month I receive scores of letters from folks who want to know one thing or another about alternative medicine. So many of these letters are of great importance and general interest that I've decided to do a section on nothing but your letters. It may not answer all your questions, but at least it's a start.

Remember, even though I can't answer all your letters, I do read them, and all of your comments, criticisms, suggestions, and even your compliments are stored in that giant computer in my head. So, being a masochist, keep those letters coming — they mean more than you could possibly know.

Q. My father is being treated for bacterial endocarditis (infection of the heart valves). He got the pneumonia shot, got pneumonia, and then it settled on his heart valves. He has been on massive doses of antibiotics for three months and they can't seem to get him well. Would the light therapy help him? — D. T., *Pennsylvania*

A. This case caught my attention because I had to wonder if there was any relationship between the pneumonia shot and the development of the heart infection. Bacterial endocarditis is not a common disease, so why did this perfectly healthy man ("walked two miles a day before he got sick") contract this serious disease?

No one knows what happens in the body when we inject foreign animal protein into it. Most of the injections are derived from animal tissues and no one really knows what the long-term consequences are because the studies simply haven't been done. I suspect that the "injectionists" are afraid of what they might find.

Florence Nightingale, among others, believed that immunizations caused a delayed effect, and that the disease, when it appeared, would be often more serious *and might, in fact, take a different form.* This case might be a good example of that phenomenon, but we can't prove it.

The light therapy D.T. refers to would be the treatment of choice but, unfortunately, it is not used in American hospitals. For more information, see my new book, Into the Light.

Q. Last summer, a 40-year-old man, supposedly in perfect health, dropped dead in the annual Peachtree Road Race in Atlanta. This seems to justify your stand that excessive exercise is dangerous to your health, especially for men over 40. Could this death have been avoided? —*W.W.W., Georgia*

A. Sudden death from excessive exercise is not uncommon in supposedly fit individuals, almost always men. *Six-mile races are not for middle-aged men.* Even young men die from exertion beyond what the human body was designed to withstand. The original Marathoner died at the finish line. Could the death have been prevented? Predictability, even with all the high technology, is poor but it seems safe to say that he probably would not have had the attack if, like me, he was observing the race on the evening news. Excessive exercise, including prolonged jogging (it seems

everywhere I look people are running with a pale, ago-
nized look on their face), isn't even safe for professional
athletes. New York Yankee catcher, Elston Howard, body
builder Charles Atlas, Paavo Nurmi, the "flying Finn,"
Olympian John Kelly, and the greatest jogger of them all,
Jim Fixx, all *died of heart attacks while jogging* — and that's
only a partial list.

What is the most common cause of death among
professional marathon runners? Heart attacks. What
chance do you have? Again, predictability is poor, but
you should know that an amazing number of professional athletes die young, so all that "fitness" can be fatal.

In addition, women run the additional risk of osteoporosis and menstrual irregularities from excessive jogging. Just because you're incredibly fit doesn't mean
you're incredibly healthy.

Most of what you have heard about stress testing for
predicting the soundness of your cardiovascular system
is wrong. The information is useless and the procedure is
dangerous. Sudden death is not uncommon during or
just after stress testing on a treadmill. If your doctor sug-
gests that you have a stress test, tell him you have a bad
knee. Angiograms, the X-rays of your heart blood vessels, are also poor predictors.

Action to Take

1. Stop endangering your health with violent exercise — you're not as young as you used to be and it may
shorten your life rather than prolong it.

2. Even if you are told by your doctor that you're in
"perfect health" (there is no such thing — nobody is perfect), I would recommend a course of chelation therapy
yearly if you are over 50 and every six months if you are
over 60. For more information on this treatment, read my
special report, "Chelation Works!"

Q. A friend of mine used to work at the University of Florida and his project was to create antibiotic-resistant gonorrhea. What would be the point of this research? Doesn't this make you wonder about the rumors that the AIDS virus was created by scientists? — *ES., Florida*

A. The answer to the second question is that it's no rumor — AIDS was created in a laboratory. I wrote this up in detail in my book, *AIDS — The End of Civilization,* now in print under the new title AIDS and Biological Warfare.

It is routine for laboratories to create antibiotic-resistant bacteria for the purpose of designing new drugs that are effective against antibiotic-resistant bugs. It is possible that some of these super germs have escaped from the laboratories. In fact, it would be hard to imagine it *not* occurring — scientists, like other humans, are prone to be careless. It would take a demented, population-control animal worshiper to do such a thing on purpose — Bertrand Russell and B.F. Skinner would be good role models — but we will not be allowed in our lifetime to know who created the AIDS virus. I have scientific contacts in Europe who claim to know and they are people of the highest integrity. It could be *dangerous* to know, especially if you have a big mouth — like me. So they will probably never tell me.

Q. I have heard that folic acid will greatly alleviate the terrible problem of menorrhagia (extreme and frequent uterine bleeding simulating heavy and frequent "periods"). Do you have an opinion on this and, if not, do you have any other suggestions? — *A.A., New Zealand*

A. I tried to find information on the use of folic acid in the treatment of menorrhagia but had no success. Often this kind of information is in obscure journals, as the major establishment ones are not interested in simple cures.

In doing the research, however, I did come up with something interesting from the South African literature. The South African researchers found that women with menorrhagia are usually deficient in vitamin A. Vitamin A is essential to the proper development of the follicle of the ovary, i.e., the remarkable little workshop that develops monthly to extrude an egg from the ovary and then turns itself into a hormone factory. Every month this little enterprise is created in one or other of the ovaries (they alternate), in hopes of catching a sperm and creating another human life — usually they are disappointed but they keep trying every month — for 40 years.

If this little hormone factory doesn't get enough vitamin A, it doesn't produce hormones properly and the menstrual cycle is disrupted — and menorrhagia, excess bleeding, may result.

This is the sort of thing that the average doctor, when asked by his patient, would say: "Oh, pish posh, what will you vitamin addicts come up with next — that's not science — it's balderdash!"

To which you should reply: "Well, Doctor, the level of endogenous 17 beta-estradiol does appear to be elevated when women with menorrhagia are treated with vitamin A and vitamin A *is* a cofactor of 3 beta-dehydrogenase steroidogenesis. So isn't it true that an A deficiency might lead to an impairment of this vital enzymatic action, thus resulting in menorrhagia?"

Then you nail him with the punch line: "At the Johannesburg General Hospital in Johannesburg, South Africa, they have used vitamin A as *standard practice* for the treatment of menorrhagia for the past ten years and have had a *92 percent* cure rate."

Anyway, after you have had your fun, go to the health food store and purchase — while you still can without a prescription — 25,000 IU vitamin A capsules and take one twice a day. If this doesn't work, add zinc, 25 mg twice daily, and vitamin E, 400 IU, twice daily. There are also scientific reasons for these additions to the therapy, when needed, but your doctor won't be interested in them, either.

Ref: *South African Medical Journal*, February 12, 1977

Q. My son is told that he cannot donate blood because he was in the Gulf War. We get various explanations: sand flea bites (which the troops were not aware of), malaria pills they took, and even a pill for prophylaxis against nerve gas. The obvious implication is that his blood is no longer healthy because of what they did to him or because of what the desert did to him. What can we do? — *MM., Pennsylvania.*

A. Unfortunately, you can do nothing. Troops, especially in a war situation, are at the mercy of their commanders — it can't be any other way. (One more in a very long list of reasons war should be the *last* resort for solving a problem.)

In a war, the invader faces two enemies: the opposing troops and the microorganisms of the region to which he may never have been exposed, and for which he therefore has no immunity. Unfortunately, a lot of useless, and sometimes dangerous, shots are given to troops because the medical corps must avoid epidemics at all costs. There are other methods for controlling epidemics, but these are seldom thought out because the mass inoculation of soldiers is the most "cost effective." Whether they actually work or not has, in most cases, never been proven.

When your son becomes ill, he should always inform the doctor that he has been in the Middle East under war conditions so that esoteric diseases can be considered in the diagnosis.

I will have more to say about this in a feature article about the Gulf War Syndrome in the near future. Please stay tuned; this one could get interesting.

Q. Can you tell me anything about a medication called "Bone Restore," which is claimed to "Build bones four times faster than calcium alone." — L.L., *California*

A. I don't usually answer questions about non-prescription health products in this column unless there is something really special about it (or especially bad about it). But this question brings up a general response about a product manufacturer making extravagant claims.

First, there is no evidence that taking elemental calcium salts will build your bones at all. So four times zero would equal zero — not an impressive result. The secret to fleshing out the truth is to write a nice letter to the company, tell them how pleased you are that they have solved this important problem and that you are going to recommend the product to your friends. But, first, would they kindly send the scientific research literature to you on which they base their marvelous product?

If you get no reply from the company or they send a generic form letter — "We are pleased that you like our Cow Lick brand of body odor depressant. Enclosed is a catalogue of our other fine products" — then that's all the answer you need.

Q. Another newsletter that I take says that osteo-porosis is caused by excessive meat in the diet. The letter says that urea and uric acid "overwork the kidneys" and that protein from animal sources is especially bad. Do you agree with this? — G.S., *Florida*

A. I do not agree at all. If it were true, then osteoporosis would be a serious problem in various tribes in Africa, such as among my friends, the Karamojong. They, and many other tribes in Africa, live on animal protein almost exclusively, and yet osteoporosis is rarely seen among them. Why would a basic food that man has been eating for thousands of years suddenly become the cause of a major health problem? There are a lot more logical answers to the osteoporosis epidemic than blaming it on Rosebud, my favorite cow. -

There appear to be three major factors involved in osteoporosis: calcium, magnesium, and phosphorus. Our modern diet has the ratios of these elements terribly deranged and the result is osteoporosis and accelerated aging. I plan to do a major piece on osteoporosis later. In the meantime, have a good steak and eat it rare.

Q. I have had all of my female organs removed and my doctor has put me on Premarin. Could this cause breast cancer? — D.K., *Illinois*

A. The controversy over estrogen (Premarin) and its possible relation to cancer rages on, and no one (including me) knows of a definite causal relationship. There is no doubt that estrogen relieves the hot flashes seen in menopause but there is no proof that it will prevent osteoporosis. Many doctors are convinced that it does; I am not. If your mother didn't have osteoporosis then you will probably not have it, either.

Q. Due to your liberating influence, I am not as paranoid about the sun as before. Because of my skin cancer history, do you have any further advice on the subject of the sun and skin cancer? — W.G.G., *Pennsylvania*

A. Yes, and I am glad you asked. In the excellent article you sent to me, from *the Journal of the American Academy of Dermatology* (JAAD), the authors discuss the possibility that *repeated* sunburning may be a factor in the type of melanoma skin cancer that you have.

It is reasonable to expect, and in fact has been proven, that severe burn trauma to the skin will have a permanent, adverse effect on the skin. However, you are not likely to catch cancer from the sun unless you are constantly in the sun for years on end. But even then, the most likely cancer would be basal cell, which is easily curable with surgery.

But we all wish to avoid aging as long as possible (I'm fighting it every step of the way — I do not intend to grow old gracefully) and clearly, excess exposure to the sun, especially sun-burning, can age the skin in susceptible people, especially blondes and redheads.

The dramatic increase in melanoma skin cancer in the last 30 years is astounding. If the current rate of increase continues, *one person in 150, born in the year 2000, will develop this kind of fatal cancer.* In not-so-sunny Scandinavia, the incidence of melanoma is doubling every seven years.

Blaming melanoma on scanty bathing suits, as suggested in the JAAD article, doesn't stand up to an analysis of the skin distribution of the disease. While it is true that on some women the bathing suit has practically disappeared (I'm not complaining, you understand), even in the most modest of times, women's bathing suits left the legs below the knees exposed to the sun. They didn't get melanoma of the lower leg because melanoma was practically unknown. But today the lower leg is the second most common site for this malignancy.

Perhaps even more convincing, the genital area in women is not an uncommon site for malignant melanoma. Even today, unless I'm attending the wrong beaches, that's one area that remains covered.

There is an interesting theory that has been around, but ignored for 20 years, which was mentioned in the JAAD article. It has to do with what the theorists call a "solar circulating factor." The idea is that some unknown factor in sunlight that enters the body and circulates to all areas of the skin, accounts for melanoma not being well-correlated with areas of sun-exposed skin.

The authors of the article reveal their bias against the sun by not pointing out that the so-called solar circulating factor could just as well be caused by constant exposure to man-made lights — an "artificial-light circulating factor." But their most glaring omission in this otherwise excellent review is their failure to discuss the light-deficiency theories of Dr. John Ott.

Dr. Ott was the first to point out that 99 percent of the lights most of us are exposed to are grossly distorted from the natural, full spectrum of sunlight. Most commercial lamps are heavy in the yellow and red end of the light spectrum and deficient in the blue, shorter wave lengths. You are receiving light energy through your eyes to your brain, and thus to the rest of your body, that is incomplete. It's like a vitamin preparation with the vitamin C removed and excess vitamin D added. The preparation is unbalanced, just as your artificial lights are unbalanced, and both types of deficiency, vitamin or light, may lead to disease — including malignant melanoma.

As you will recall from my writings and the article that you sent to me, it's the *office* workers in sunny Queensland, Australia, who have the highest incidence of melanoma, not people such as lifeguards, who are in the sun most of every day. The office workers are starving in the midst of plenty of natural light, right outside their windows.

Finally, here is the "further advice" that you asked for:

1. Don't be paranoid about the sun. I think we have cured you of that.

2. Install full-spectrum lights in your home. You can obtain full-spectrum lights from Health Lighting, at 800-557-5127.

3. Avoid severe sunburn but remember that Old Sol is the key to life on earth. The Creator placed us at just the right distance from the sun to enable the earth to flourish with plants, animals — and dermatologists.

Ref: *Journal of the American Academy of Dermatologists*, October 1984.

About Doctor William Campbell Douglass II

Dr. Douglass reveals medical truths, and deceptions, often at risk of being labeled heretical. He is consumed by a passion for living a long healthy life, and wants his readers to share that passion. Their health and well-being comes first. He is anti-dogmatic, and unwavering in his dedication to improve the quality of life of his readers. He has been called "the conscience of modern medicine," a "medical maverick," and has been voted "Doctor of the Year" by the National Health Federation. His medical experiences are far reaching-from battling malaria in Central America - to fighting deadly epidemics at his own health clinic in Africa - to flying with U.S. Navy crews as a flight surgeon - to working for 10 years in emergency medicine here in the States. These learning experiences, not to mention his keen storytelling ability and wit, make Dr. Douglass' newsletters (Daily Dose and Real Health) and books uniquely interesting and fun to read. He shares his no-frills, no-bull approach to health care, often amazing his readers by telling them to ignore many widely-hyped good-health practices (like staying away from red meat, avoiding coffee, and eating like a bird), and start living again by eating REAL food, taking some inexpensive supplements, and doing the pleasurable things that make life livable. Readers get all this, plus they learn how to burn fat, prevent cancer, boost libido, and so much more. And, Dr. Douglass is not afraid to challenge the latest studies that come out, and share the real story with his readers. Dr. William C. Douglass has led a colorful, rebellious, and crusading life. Not many physicians would dare put their professional reputations on the line as many times as this courageous healer has. A vocal opponent of "business-as-usual" medicine, Dr. Douglass has championed patients' rights and physician commitment to wellness throughout his career. This dedicated physician has repeatedly gone far beyond the call of duty in his work to spread the truth about alternative therapies. For a full year, he endured economic and physical hardship to work with physicians at the Pasteur Institute in St. Petersburg, Russia, where advanced research on photoluminescence was being conducted. Dr. Douglass comes from a distinguished family of physicians. He is the fourth generation Douglass to practice medicine, and his son is also a physician. Dr. Douglass graduated from the University of Rochester, the Miami School of Medicine, and the Naval School of Aviation and Space Medicine.

You want to protect those you love from the health dangers the authorities aren't telling you about, and learn the incredible cures that they've scorned and ignored?
Subscribe to the free Daily Dose updates "...the straight scoop about health, medicine, and politics." by sending an e-mail to real_sub@agoramail.net with the word "subscribe" in the subject line.

Dr. William Campbell Douglass'
Real Health:

Had Enough?

Enough turkey burgers and sprouts?

Enough forcing gallons of water down your throat?

Enough exercising until you can barely breathe?

Before you give up everything just because "everyone" says it's healthy...

Learn the facts from Dr. William Campbell Douglass, medicine's most acclaimed myth-buster. In every issue of Dr. Douglass' Real Health newsletter, you'll learn shocking truths about "junk medicine" and how to stay healthy while eating eggs, meat and other foods you love.

With the tips you'll receive from Real Health, you'll see your doctor less, spend a lot less money and be happier and healthier while you're at it. The road to Real Health is actually easier, cheaper and more pleasant than you dared to dream.

Subscribe to Real Health today by calling 1-800-981-7162 or visit the Real Health web site at www.realhealthnews.com.
Use promotional code : DRHBDZZZ

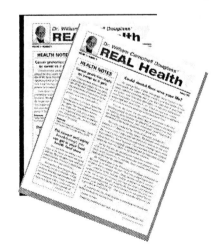

If you knew of a procedure that could save thousand. maybe millions, of people dying from AIDS, cancer, and other dreaded killers....

Would you cover it up?

It's unthinkable that what could be the best solution ever to stopping the world's killer diseases is being ignored, scorned, and rejected. But that is exactly what's happening right now.

The procedure is called "photoluminescence". It's a thoroughly tested, proven therapy that uses the healing power of the light to perform almost miraculous cures.

This remarkable treatment works its incredible cures by stimulating the body's own immune responses. That's why it cures so many ailments--and why it's been especially effective against AIDS! Yet, 50 years ago, it virtually disappeared from the halls of medicine.

Why has this incredible cure been ignored by the medical authorities of this country? You'll find the shocking answer here in the pages of this new edition of Into the Light. Now available with the blood irradiation Instrument Diagram and a complete set of instructions for building your own "Treatment Device". Also includes details on how to use this unique medical instrument.

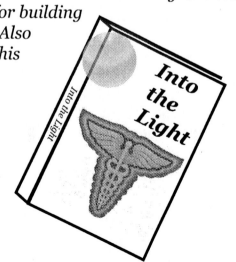

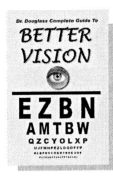

Dr. Douglass' Complete Guide to Better Vision

A report about eyesight and what can be done to improve it naturally. But I've also included information about how the eye works, brief descriptions of various common eye conditions, traditional remedies to eye problems, and a few simple suggestions that may help you maintain your eyesight for years to come. -William Campbell Douglass II, MD

The Hypertension Report. Say Good Bye to High Blood Pressure.

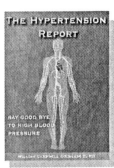

An estimated 50 million Americans have high blood pressure. Often called the "silent killer" because it may not cause symptoms until the patient has suffered serious damage to the arterial system. Diet, exercise, potassium supplements chelation therapy and practically anything but drugs is the way to go and alternatives are discussed in this report.

Grandma Bell's A To Z Guide To Healing With Herbs.

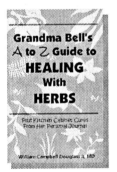

This book is all about - coming home. What I once believed to be old wives' tales - stories long destroyed by the new world of science - actually proved to be the best treatment for many of the common ailments you and I suffer through. So I put a few of them together in this book with the sincere hope that Grandma Bell's wisdom will help you recover your common sense, and take responsibility for your own health. -William Campbell Douglass II, MD

Prostate Problems: Safe, Simple, Effective Relief for Men over 50.

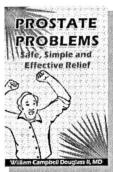

Don't be frightened into surgery or drugs you may not need. First, get the facts about prostate problems... know all your options, so you can make the best decisions. This fully documented report explains the dangers of conventional treatments, and gives you alternatives that could save you more than just money!

Color me Healthy
The Healing Powers of Colors

"He's crazy!"
"He's got to be a quack!"
"Who gave this guy his medical license?"
"He's a nut case!"

In case you're wondering, those are the reactions you'll probably get if you show your doctor this report. I know the idea of healing many common ailments simply by exposing them to colored light sounds far-fetched, but when you see the evidence, you'll agree that color is truly an amazing medical breakthrough.

When I first heard the stories, I reacted much the same way. But the evidence so convinced me, that I had to try color therapy in my practice. My results were truly amazing.

-William Campbell Douglass II, MD

Order your complete set of Roscolene filters (choice of 3 sizes) to be used with the "Color Me Healthy" therapy. The eleven Roscolene filters are # 809, 810, 818, 826, 828, 832, 859, 861, 866, 871, and 877. The filters come with protective separator sheets between each filter. The color names and the Roscolene filter(s) used to produce that particular color, are printed on a card included with the filters and a set of instructions on how to fit them to a lamp.

Rhino Publishing
www.rhinopublish.com

What Is Going on Here?

Peroxides are supposed to be bad for you. Free radicals and all that. But now we hear that hydrogen peroxide is good for us. Hydrogen peroxide will put extra oxygen in your blood. There's no doubt about that. Hydrogen peroxide costs pennies. So if you can get oxygen into the blood cheaply and safely, maybe cancer (which doesn't like oxygen), emphysema, AIDS, and many other terrible diseases can be treated effectively. Intravenous hydrogen peroxide rapidly relieves allergic reactions, influenza symptoms, and acute viral infections.

No one expects to live forever. But we would all like to have a George Burns finish. The prospect of finishing life in a nursing home after abandoning your tricycle in the mobile home park is not appealing. Then comes the loss of control of vital functions the ultimate humiliation. Is life supposed to be from tricycle to tricycle and diaper to diaper? You come into this world crying, but do you have to leave crying? I don't believe you do. And you won't either after you see the evidence. Sounds too good to be true, doesn't it? Read on and decide for yourself.

-William Campbell Douglass II, MD

Rhino Publishing S.A.
www.rhinopublish.com

HYDROGEN PEROXIDE

Medical Miracle

H₂O

Don't drink your milk!

If you knew what we know about milk... BLEECHT! All that pasteurization, homogenization and processing is not only cooking all the nutrients right out of your favorite drink. It's also adding toxic levels of vitamin D.

This fascinating book tells the whole story about milk. How it once was nature's perfect food...how "raw," unprocessed milk can heal and boost your immune system ... why you can't buy it legally in this country anymore, and what we could do to change that.

Dr. "Douglass traveled all over the world, tasting all kinds of milk from all kinds of cows, poring over dusty research books in ancient libraries far from home, to write this light-hearted but scientifically sound book.

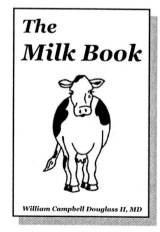

The
Milk Book

William Campbell Douglass II, MD

Rhino Publishing, S.A.
www.rhinopublish.com

Eat Your Cholesterol!
Eat Meat, Drink Milk, Spread The Butter- And Live Longer!
How to Live off the Fat of the Land and Feel Great.

Americans are being saturated with anti-cholesterol propaganda. If you watch very much television, you're probably one of the millions of Americans who now has a terminal case of cholesterol phobia. The propaganda is relentless and is often designed to produce fear and loathing of this worst of all food contaminants. You never hear the food propagandists bragging about their product being fluoride-free or aluminum-free, two of our truly serious food-additive problems. But cholesterol, an essential nutrient, not proven to be harmful in any quantity, is constantly pilloried as a menace to your health. If you don't use corn oil, Fleischmann's margarine, and Egg Beaters, you're going straight to atherosclerosis hell with stroke, heart attack, and premature aging -- and so are your kids. Never feel guilty about what you eat again! Dr. Douglass shows you why red meat, eggs, and dairy products aren't the dietary demons we're told they are. But beware: This scientifically sound report goes against all the "common wisdom" about the foods you should eat. Read with an open mind.

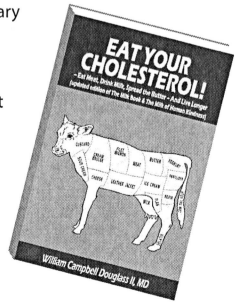

Rhino Publishing, S.A.
www.rhinopublish.com

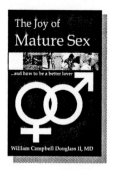

The Joy of Mature Sex and How to Be a Better Lover

Humans are very confused about what makes good sex. But I believe humans have more to offer each other than this total licentiousness common among animals. We're talking about mature sex. The kind of sex that made this country great.

Stop Aging or Slow the Process How Exercise With Oxygen Therapy (EWOT) Can Help

EWOT (pronounced ee-watt) stands for Exercise With Oxygen Therapy. This method of prolonging your life is so simple and you can do it at home at a minimal cost. When your cells don't get enough oxygen, they degenerate and die and so you degenerate and die. It's as simple as that.

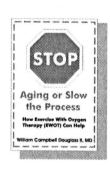

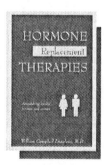

Hormone Replacement Therapies: Astonishing Results For Men And Women

It is accurate to say that when the endocrine glands start to fail, you start to die. We are facing a sea change in longevity and health in the elderly. Now, with the proper supplemental hormones, we can slow the aging process and, in many cases, reverse some of the signs and symptoms of aging.

Add 10 Years to Your Life With some "best of" Dr. Douglass' writings.

To add ten years to your life, you need to have the right attitude about health and an understanding of the health industry and what it's feeding you. Following the established line on many health issues could make you very sick or worse! Achieve dynamic health with this collection of some of the "best of" Dr. Douglass' newsletters.

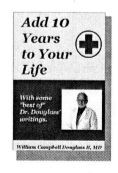

How did AIDS become one of the Greatest Biological Disasters in the History of Mankind?

GET THE FACTS

AIDS and BIOLOGICAL WARFARE covers the history of plagues from the past to today's global confrontation with AIDS, the Prince of Plagues. Completely documented *AIDS and BIOLOGICAL WARFARE* helps you make your own decisions about how to survive in a world ravaged by this horrible plague.

You will learn that AIDS is not a naturally occuring disease process as you have been led to believe, but a man-made biological nightmare that has been unleashed and is now threatening the very existence of human life on the planet.

There is a smokescreen of misinformation clouding the AIDS issue. Now, for the first time, learn the truth about the nature of the crisis our planet faces: its origin -- how AIDS is really transmited and alternatives for treatment. Find out what they are not telling you about AIDS and Biological Warfare, and how to protect yourself and your loved ones. AIDS is a serious problem worldwide, but it is no longer the major threat. You need to know the whole story. To protect yourself, you must know the truth about biological warfare.

PAINFUL DILEMMA

Are we fighting the wrong war?

We are spending millions on the war against drugs while we
should be fighting the war against pain with those drugs!

As you will read in this book, the war on drugs was lost a long time ago and,
when it comes to the war against pain, pain is winning! An article in USA Today
(11/20/02) reveals that dying patients are not getting relief from pain. It seems
the doctors are torn between fear of the government, certainly justified, and a
clinging to old and out dated ideas about pain, which is NOT justified.

A group called Last Acts, a coalition of health-care groups, has released a very
discouraging study of all 50 states that nearly half of the 1.6 million Americans
living in nursing homes suffer from untreated pain. They said that life was being
extended but it amounted to little more than "extended pain and suffering."

This book offers insight into the history of pain treatment and the current failed
philosophies of contemporary medicine. Plus it describes some of today's most
advanced treatments for alleviating certain kinds of pain. This book is not another
"self-help" book touting home remedies; rather, Painful Dilemma: Patients in
Pain -- People in Prison, takes a hard look at where we've gone wrong and what
we (you) can do to help a loved one who is living with chronic pain.

The second half of this book is a must read if you value your freedom. We now
have the ridiculous and tragic situation of people
in pain living in a government-created hell by
restriction of narcotics and people in prison for
trying to bring pain relief by the selling of
narcotics to the suffering. The end result of the
"war on drugs" has been to create the greatest
and most destructive cartel in history, so great,
in fact, that the drug Mafia now controls most
of the world economy.

Rhino Publishing S.A.
www.rhinopublish.com

Live the Adventure!

Why would anyone in their right mind put everything they own in storage and move to Russia, of all places?! But when maverick physician Bill Douglass left a profitable medical practice in a peaceful mountaintop town to pursue "pure medical truth".... none of us who know him well was really surprised.

After All, anyone who's braved the outermost reaches of darkest Africa, the mean streets of Johannesburg and New York, and even a trip to Washington to testify before the Senate, wouldn't bat and eye at ducking behind the Iron Curtain for a little medical reconnaissance!

Enjoy this imaginative, funny, dedicated man's tales of wonder and woe as he treks through a year in St. Petersburg, working on a cure for the world's killer diseases. We promise --

YOU WON'T BE BORED!

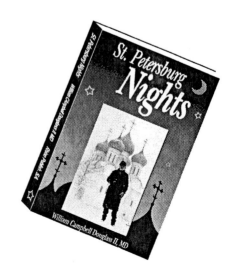

Rhino Publishing S.A.
www.rhinopublish.com

THE SMOKER'S PARADOX
THE HEALTH BENEFITS OF TOBACCO!

The benefits of smoking tobacco have been common knowledge for centuries. From sharpening mental acuity to maintaining optimal weight, the relatively small risks of smoking have always been outweighed by the substantial improvement to mental and physical health. Hysterical attacks on tobacco notwithstanding, smokers always weigh the good against the bad and puff away or quit according to their personal preferences. Now the same anti-tobacco enterprise that has spent billions demonizing the pleasure of smoking is providing additional reasons to smoke. Alzheimer's, Parkinson's, Tourette's Syndrome, even schizophrenia and cocaine addiction are disorders that are alleviated by tobacco. Add in the still inconclusive indication that tobacco helps to prevent colon and prostate cancer and the endorsement for smoking tobacco by the medical establishment is good news for smokers and non-smokers alike. Of course the revelation that tobacco is good for you is ruined by the pharmaceutical industry's plan to substitute the natural and relatively inexpensive tobacco plant with their overpriced and ineffective nicotine substitutions. Still, when all is said and done, the positive revelations regarding tobacco are very good reasons indeed to keep lighting those cigars - but only 4 a day!

THE SMOKER'S PARADOX

William Campbell Douglass II, MD

The health benefits of tobacco

Rhino Publishing, S.A
www.rhinopublish.com

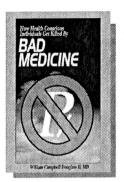

Bad Medicine
How Individuals Get Killed By Bad Medicine.

Do you really need that new prescription or that overnight stay in the hospital? In this report, Dr. Douglass reveals the common medical practices and misconceptions endangering your health. Best of all, he tells you the pointed (but very revealing!) questions your doctor prays you never ask. Interesting medical facts about popular remedies are revealed.

Dangerous Legal Drugs
The Poisons in Your Medicine Chest.

If you knew what we know about the most popular prescription and over-the-counter drugs, you'd be sick. That's why Dr. Douglass wrote this shocking report about the poisons in your medicine chest. He gives you the low-down on different categories of drugs. Everything from painkillers and cold remedies to tranquilizers and powerful cancer drugs.

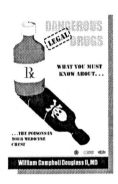

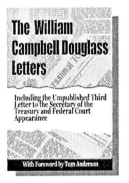

The William Campbell Douglass Letters.
Expose of Government Machinations
(Vietnam War).

THE WILLIAM CAMPBELL DOUGLASS LETTERS. Dr. Douglass' Defense in 1968 Tax Case and Expose of Government Machinations during the Vietnam War.

The Eagle's Feather. A Novel of
International Political Intrigue.

Although The Eagle's Feather is a work of fiction set in the 1970's, it is built, as with most fiction, on a framework of plausibility and background information. This is a fiction book that could not have been written were it not for various ominous aspects, which pose a clear and present danger to the security of the United States.

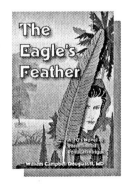

Rhino Publishing

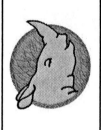

ORDER FORM

PURCHASER INFORMATION

Purchaser's Name (Please Print): _____

Shipping Address (Do not use a P.O. Box): _____

City: _____ State/Prov.: _____ Country: _____

Zip/Postal Code: _____ Telephone No.: _____ Fax No.: _____

E-Mail Address (if interested in receiving free e-Books when available): _____

CREDIT CARD INFO (CIRCLE ONE):

MASTERCARD, VISA, AMERICAN EXPRESS, DISCOVER, JCB, DINER'S CLUB, CARTE BLANCHE.

Charge my Card -> Number #: _____ Exp.: _____

*Security Code: _____ * Required for all MasterCard, Visa and American Express purchases. For your security, we require that you enter your card's verification number. The verification number is also called a CCV number. This code is the 3 digits farthest right in the signature field on the back of your VISA/MC, or the 4 digits to the right on the front of your American Express card. Your credit card statement will show a **different name than Rhino Publishing** as the vendor.

WE DO NOT share your private information, we use 3ʳᵈ party credit card processing service to process your order only.

ADDITIONAL INFORMATION

If your shipping address is not the same as your credit card billing address, please indicate your card billing address here.

_____   Type of card: _____

Name on the card

Billing Address: _____

City: _____   State/Prov.: _____   Zip/Postal Code: _____

Fax a copy of this order to:
RHINO PUBLISHING, S.A.

1-888-317-6767 or International #: + 416-352-5126

To order by mail, send your payment by first class mail only to the following address. Please include a copy of this order form. Make your check or bank drafts (NO postal money order) payable to RHINO PUBLISHING, S.A. and mail to:

Rhino Publishing, S.A.
Attention: PTY 5048
P.O. Box 025724
Miami, FL.
USA 33102

Digital E-books also available online: www.rhinopublish.com

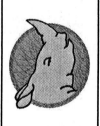

Rhino
Publishing

ORDER
FORM

Purchaser's Name (Please Print):

I would like to order the following paperback book of Dr. Douglass (Alternative Medicine Books):

___	X	9962-636-04-3	Add 10 Years to Your Life. With some "best of" Dr. Douglass writings.	$13.99 $ ___
___	X	9962-636-07-8	AIDS and Biological Warfare. What They Are Not Telling You!	$17.99 $ ___
___	X	9962-636-09-4	Bad Medicine. How Individuals Get Killed By Bad Medicine.	$11.99 $ ___
___	X	9962-636-10-8	Color Me Healthy. The Healing Power of Colors.	$11.99 $ ___
___	X	9962-636 -XX-X	Color Filters for Color Me Healthy. 11 Basic Roscolene Filters for Lamps.	$21.89 $ ___
___	X	9962-636-15-9	Dangerous Legal Drugs. The Poisons in Your Medicine Chest.	$13.99 $ ___
___	X	9962-636-18-3	Dr. Douglass' Complete Guide to Better Vision. Improve eyesight naturally.	$11.99 $ ___
___	X	9962-636-19-1	Eat Your Cholesterol! How to Live off the Fat of the Land and Feel Great.	$11.99 $ ___
___	X	9962-636-12-4	Grandma Bell's A To Z Guide To Healing. Her Kitchen Cabinet Cures.	$14.99 $ ___
___	X	9962-636-22-1	Hormone Replacement Therapies. Astonishing Results For Men & Women	$11.99 $ ___
___	X	9962-636-25-6	Hydrogen Peroxide: One of the Most Underused Medical Miracle.	$15.99 $ ___
___	X	9962-636-27-2	Into the Light. New Edition with Blood Irradiation Instrument Instructions.	$19.99 $ ___
___	X	9962-636-54-X	Milk Book. The Classic on the Nutrition of Milk and How to Benefit from it.	$17.99 $ ___

__ X __	9962-636-00-0	Painful Dilemma - Patients in Pain - People in Prison.	$17.99 $ ____
__ X __	9962-636-32-9	Prostate Problems. Safe, Simple, Effective Relief for Men over 50.	$11.99 $ ____
__ X __	9962-636-34-5	St. Petersburg Nights. Enlightening Story of Life and Science in Russia.	$17.99 $ ____
__ X __	9962-636-37-X	Stop Aging or Slow the Process. Exercise With Oxygen Therapy Can Help.	$11.99 $ ____
__ X __	9962-636-60-4	The Hypertension Report. Say Good Bye to High Blood Pressure.	$11.99 $ ____
__ X __	9962-636-48-5	The Joy of Mature Sex and How to Be a Better Lover...	$13.99 $ ____
__ X __	9962-636-43-4	The Smoker's Paradox: Health Benefits of Tobacco.	$14.99 $ ____

Political Books:

__ X __	9962-636-40-X	The Eagle's Feather. A 70's Novel of International Political Intrigue.	$15.99 $ ____
__ X __	9962-636-46-9	The W. C. D. Letters. Expose of Government Machinations (Vietnam War).	$11.99 $ ____
		SUB-TOTAL:	$ ____

____	ADD $5.00 HANDLING FOR YOUR ORDER:	$ 5.00 $ 5.00
__ X __	ADD $2.50 SHIPPING FOR EACH ITEM ON ORDER:	$ 2.50 $ ____
	NOTE THAT THE MINIMUM SHIPPING AND HANDLING IS $7.50 FOR 1 BOOK ($5.00 + $2.50)	
	For order shipped outside the US, add $5.00 per item	
__ X __	ADD $5.00 S. & H. OR EACH ITEM ON ORDER (INTERNATIONAL ORDERS ONLY)	$ 5.00 $ ____
	Allow up to 21 days for delivery (we will call you about back orders if any)	
	TOTAL:	$ ____

Fax a copy of this order to: 1-888-317-6767 or Int'l + 416-352-5126
or mail to: Rhino Publishing, S.A. Attention: PTY 5048 P.O. Box 025724, Miami, FL., 33102 USA
Digital E-books also available online: www.rhinopublish.com

Printed in the United States
44807LVS00006B/451-462

9 789962 636045